the**facts**

Muscular dystrophy

the facts

Muscular
dystrophy

THIRD EDITION

ALAN E. H. EMERY

Emeritus Professor of Human Genetics
University of Edinburgh, and
Chief Scientific Advisor
European Neuromuscular Centre

OXFORD
UNIVERSITY PRESS

OXFORD

UNIVERSITY PRESS

Great Clarendon Street, Oxford OX2 6DP

Oxford University Press is a department of the University of Oxford.
It furthers the University's objective of excellence in research, scholarship,
and education by publishing worldwide in

Oxford New York

Auckland Cape Town Dar es Salaam Hong Kong Karachi
Kuala Lumpur Madrid Melbourne Mexico City Nairobi
New Delhi Shanghai Taipei Toronto

With offices in

Argentina Austria Brazil Chile Czech Republic France Greece
Guatemala Hungary Italy Japan Poland Portugal Singapore
South Korea Switzerland Thailand Turkey Ukraine Vietnam

Oxford is a registered trade mark of Oxford University Press
in the UK and in certain other countries

Published in the United States
by Oxford University Press Inc., New York

© Oxford University Press, 2008

The moral rights of the author has been asserted
Database right Oxford University Press (maker)

First edition published 1994
Reprinted published 1996

Second edition published 2000
Reprinted published 2004

Translations of previous editions of this book are available in
French, Japanese, Ukrainian and Spanish

All rights reserved. No part of this publication may be reproduced, stored in a retrieval system,
or transmitted, in any form or by any means, without the prior permission in writing of Oxford
University Press, or as expressly permitted by law, or under terms agreed with the appropriate
reprographics rights organization. Enquiries concerning reproduction outside the scope of the
above should be sent to the Rights Department, Oxford University Press, at the address above

You must not circulate this book in any other binding or cover
and you must impose this same condition on any acquirer

British Library Cataloguing in Publication Data

Data available

Library of Congress Cataloguing in Publication Data

Data available

ISBN 978-0-19-954216-1 (Pbk.)

10 9 8 7 6 5 4 3 2 1

Typeset in Plantin
by Cepha Imaging Pvt. Ltd., Bangalore, India
Printed in Great Britain
on acid-free paper by
Clays Ltd, Bungay, Suffolk, UK

While every effort has been to ensure that the contents of this book are as complete, accurate
and up-to-date as possible at the date of writing, Oxford University Press is not able to give any
guarantee or assurance that such is the case. Readers are urged to take appropriately qualified
medical advice in all cases. The information in this book is intended to be useful to the general
reader, but should not be used as a means of self-diagnosis or for the prescription of medication.

Contents

Preface to the third edition

It is now 14 years since the first edition of this little book was published. Like many other medical conditions, particularly those like the muscular dystrophies which are genetic in causation, recent research has revealed many new facts. Apart from the more frequent forms of muscular dystrophy, such as Duchenne muscular dystrophy, many newer forms have been recognized and their genes identified. This information offers therefore more opportunities for reliable counselling in these conditions and, where appropriate, prenatal diagnosis. But perhaps the most significant advances have been in regard to new approaches to gene therapy that are now beginning to be the subject of clinical trials. Furthermore, increasing numbers of medical scientists believe new approaches through stem cell therapy may prove effective. I have attempted to discuss these various developments without excess detail. More information on such matters, as well as those of a more general nature, can be found in the list of further reading at the end of the book.

I should like to thank all those affected by muscular dystrophy and their relatives, who have offered me much useful advice. I am most grateful to Mr Philip Butcher, the Executive Director of the Muscular Dystrophy Campaign, and his colleagues who have been especially helpful in providing much useful information of practical help to patients and their families. I must also thank Oxford University Press for their encouragement and support, which as ever is very much appreciated. Finally, I must also thank my wife Marcia for her continued help in preparing the manuscript.

As in the past all royalties earned from the sale of this book are donated to support research and education into neuromuscular disorders, especially muscular dystrophy.

A.E.H.E. 2008

Preface to the second edition

It is now 6 years since the first edition of this little book appeared. In the interim, research has revealed a great many new facts about the muscular dystrophies. For example, the genes for almost all types of dystrophy have now been identified so that genetic counselling has become much more precise and prenatal diagnosis is now a real possibility for those who wish. Furthermore, there has been increasing interest and research into gene therapy. Much of this work has so far centred on animal studies and at the time of writing it is still some way from being offered to affected individuals. However, some scientists now feel that this approach to treatment may well become a reality before too long.

I should like to thank all those patients and their relatives as well as researchers who have offered me much useful advice in preparing this new edition. I must also thank my wife, Marcia, for her unstinting help in preparing the manuscript and tracing important references, and the staff of Oxford University Press for their continued support and encouragement.

A. E. H. E.

January 2000

Preface to the first edition

This little book has been written specifically for those with muscular dystrophy and their families in the hope that it will provide answers to some of the many questions which often arise with this group of diseases. In recent years research has revealed much about the cause of muscular dystrophy and opened up new approaches to possible treatment. In fact at no time in the history of the subject have the prospects for an effective treatment seemed better. I have tried to present some of these findings in terms which anyone interested will be able to appreciate. Questions relating to exercise, physiotherapy, surgery, and the psychological effects of the disease are discussed as well as problems of schooling and choice of employment. Since all the dystrophies are genetic, the ways in which the various forms are inherited and their possible prevention are also discussed. Finally, the importance of professional organizations and voluntary support groups is emphasized since these can play an important role in helping to overcome feelings of isolation which are all too frequent.

The hope is that you may find answers to some of the many problems which often have to be faced, though I am well aware that not everything can be learnt from a book! Nothing can really replace the advice and help of an experienced and sympathetic doctor, physiotherapist, nurse, or counsellor.

All royalties earned from the sale of this book will be donated to Green College, Oxford, to support medical research and education.

A. E. H. E.

May 1994

1

Introduction

If you have muscular dystrophy, or you have an affected son or daughter or other affected relative, the first thing to remember is that you are not alone and that there are many others who are similarly affected and share the same worries and concerns. Muscular dystrophy or, more accurately, the muscular dystrophies, as there are many different types, are not uncommon. There are nearly 70 000 individuals affected with a *severe form* of dystrophy in the various countries of western Europe and *at least* 40 000 in the USA. It has no predilection for any particular group of individuals but affects all races, all strata of society, and occurs throughout the world. Why then is it not more obvious? The simplest answer is that those with a physical disability often avoid society and, moreover, are often avoided by society. Furthermore, in most forms of dystrophy the resulting disability may not be obvious to the casual observer, and affected individuals often become quite adept at disguising their problems. However, for whatever reason, muscular dystrophy has, for a long time, been a neglected subject. It began to reach public awareness as a result of television programmes specifically organized for this purpose, such as the Muscular Dystrophy Campaign's Annual Meeting in Britain, the Jerry Lewis TV appeal in the USA, and Télethon in France and Italy. All of these raise a great deal of money each year for research and for the treatment of dystrophy.

Now at last society is beginning to recognize and appreciate more and more the problems of physical disability that are often caused by dystrophy. This has been partly due to media coverage but also to major advances in scientific medicine in the last few years. For a very long time, and certainly since I first became interested in the subject nearly 50 years ago, there was a general feeling of powerlessness on the part of the medical profession to deal with a problem that seemed intractable. The dystrophies were recognized as being genetic but there was no way of knowing who carried the gene until perhaps they became affected. And approaches to treatment were often 'stabs in the dark' because their cause was quite unknown.

1

This is now all changing. For the very first time we are beginning to understand the fundamental causes of these disorders and to unravel their complex biochemistry. Furthermore, and most importantly, these findings are beginning to focus the attention of physicians on *rational approaches to treatment*, which are based on the cause of the disease and therefore are much more likely to be effective. The possibility of some form of *gene therapy* is also increasingly attracting the attention of researchers.

Thus the important things to remember are that you are not alone, and that there are now good reasons for entertaining cautious optimism that effective treatments for these distressing conditions will be found in the not too distant future.

2

What is muscular dystrophy?

→ Key points

♦ The muscular dystrophies are a group of inherited diseases in which various genes controlling muscle function are defective.

♦ In most forms of dystrophy the basic underlying protein defect is now known (a deficiency of the muscle protein dystrophin in Duchenne muscular dystrophy, for example).

♦ Scientists are beginning to understand how muscle weakness develops, though many questions still remain to be answered, not least being why some people become more severely affected than others in the same family. Nevertheless, the nature of these diseases is now better understood than at any other time in the history of the subject.

One fact has been quite clear right from the very beginning, when dystrophy was first recognized as a disease entity over a hundred years ago: it is *not infectious or contagious in any way*. It cannot be spread by contact from one affected person to another, nor from household pets. Some readers might think that it is unnecessary to stress this point, but I have known patients who seemed quite convinced that they had 'caught' the disease from a relative. This is not so. Furthermore, there is no evidence that anything you do in your everyday life can cause the disease or bring it on. *All dystrophies are genetic and are due to defects in the genes*. But what does this mean? Before we can discuss details of the disease any further, it is necessary to consider a little basic science.

The genes

We are each born with certain characteristics or traits that are inherent. That is why we resemble our relatives more than we resemble others. These inherited traits are part of our constitution and include, for example, eye colour and blood groups. These traits are determined by *genes*.

All life starts off as a single cell, the fertilized egg or ovum, which then undergoes repeated divisions, ultimately to produce all the cells, tissues, and organs of the body. Each cell contains a nucleus that, when cells are treated with an appropriate dye and then viewed down the microscope, appears as a darkly stained structure within the cell (Fig. 2.1). In each nucleus there are 46 thread-like bodies called *chromosomes*, 23 of which are derived from one parent and 23 from the other. Each of these 23 chromosomes can now be individually identified because each has a particular banding pattern when stained with certain dyes. The arrangement of the chromosomes in a standard manner is referred to as a *karyotype* (Chapter 8).

The chromosomes carry the genes, and the same genes are present in every cell of the body—although only certain genes are active in particular tissues or organs. For example, a gene making muscle protein is active only in muscle tissue and a gene making haemoglobin, the oxygen-carrying chemical in red blood cells, is only active in blood-forming cells. Estimates vary, but there are probably about 30 000 genes in each nucleus. We still know very little about the many genes that determine and control such common traits as intelligence, stature, and our general 'appearance'. Oddly, we know more about genes that result in diseases such as dystrophy (Chapter 8).

Genes are composed of *DNA* (deoxyribonucleic acid), a complicated double-stranded molecule (called a double helix) in which is coded the information for making amino acids and proteins, essential components of our bodies. DNA is composed of four bases (abbreviated to C, T, A, G). Any combination of three bases specifies or codes for different amino acids. The amino acids so produced then join up to form a particular protein or part of a protein. The simplest way to visualize the cause of dystrophy is to imagine that normally a particular gene makes (synthesizes) a protein essential for normal muscle activity. However, if this gene changes, a change that we refer to as a *mutation*, then the gene either does not synthesize the protein or synthesizes an abnormal protein so that the muscle no longer functions properly. Though X-rays and certain chemicals are known to cause mutations in animals, the cause of the vast majority of mutations in humans is at present quite unknown. They seem to occur randomly, and the mutation that causes dystrophy in a family

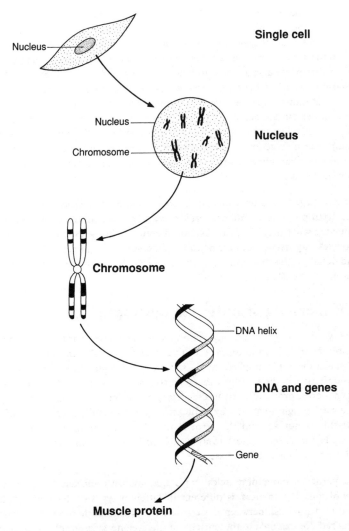

Single cell

Nucleus

Nucleus

Nucleus

Chromosome

Nucleus

Chromosome

DNA helix

DNA and genes

Gene

Muscle protein

Figure 2.1 Diagram of the relationship between the cell nucleus, chromosomes, DNA, and genes.

appears to be a purely chance event. Certainly we have no explanation for why dystrophy should originate in one family rather than another. In some families the mutant gene that causes the disease can be traced back several generations. In others, the causative mutation occurs in the egg or sperm that led to that particular affected individual. These and related matters will be discussed later in Chapter 8. How we can tell which gene is abnormal out of several thousand is the province of *molecular genetics*. The most important development in the subject, whereby abnormal genes can be identified and traced in families and even shown to be present in the fetus while still in the womb, began some 20 years ago. In fact, Duchenne muscular dystrophy was the very first condition in which a disease-producing gene was identified using these techniques.

We now have laboratory tools that have allowed us to identify genes for various dystrophies, to isolate such genes, and then to determine what they do. Knowing what they do normally, and therefore what goes wrong in disease, provides important clues for possible treatments. The interested reader can find details of this new and important science in several modern texts listed at the end of the book.

The meaning of 'muscular dystrophy'

The word *dystrophy* originally comes from two Greek words: *dys*, meaning abnormal or faulty, and *trophe*, meaning food or nourishment. Thus the term muscular dystrophy implied that in some way the nourishment of the muscle was defective, in the same way that a person who does not eat the correct food will not grow properly. Early in the history of the subject the defect in the disease was thought in some way to be actually due to faulty muscle 'nutrition'. But this is not so, and the term is therefore something of a misnomer. Nowadays it is used to indicate abnormal muscle wasting and weakness, which are the hallmarks of the disease.

The particular group of muscles that is predominantly affected, or the *distribution* of muscle weakness, is different in different types of dystrophy, and is used to distinguish between these types. In some, muscle weakness remains localized, for example to the muscles of the eye and face. In others the major muscle groups responsible for moving the limbs become mainly involved, and later other muscles may also become affected. But whatever the particular type of dystrophy, the essential feature is muscle wasting and weakness.

Muscular dystrophy

This term includes many conditions presenting with muscle wasting and weakness. All are genetic, but different types are due to different genes and differ in severity.

There are many different causes of muscle wasting and weakness apart from dystrophy, which the physician must first exclude when making the diagnosis. These other causes are not all genetic. For example, muscle weakness may result from a disease that affects the nerve supply to the muscle. A common cause for this in the past was poliomyelitis, but there are also some inherited diseases where this may occur. Muscular dystrophy, however, does *not* result from a disease of the muscle's nerve supply. It is a disease that *primarily* affects muscle tissue, though in some dystrophies other tissues and organs may also be affected.

Muscle weakness

The muscle weakness that occurs in all types of dystrophy has certain features in common. It is usually *symmetrical*, i.e. the weakness on the two sides of the body is often very similar, though one side may sometimes *seem* more affected than the other. Thus, a right-handed person may be more aware of weakness in that arm, though careful testing by the physician may well reveal a similar degree of weakness in both arms. The weakness is usually *progressive*, though this again differs very much from one type of dystrophy to another. Some types begin in infancy or early childhood and may be severe and progress rapidly, but others coming on in later life may be very mild. There is often quite a lot of variation between different affected people with the same type of dystrophy, even within the same family, and some may be concerned because they are more severely affected than a relative of the same age. We are just beginning to understand how this can occur in myotonic dystrophy, for example, but it has to be admitted that in other dystrophies we still have no satisfactory explanation to offer for such variation in families. On the other hand, in some types of dystrophy, such as Duchenne muscular dystrophy, the course of the disease is fairly uniform and does not usually vary a great deal.

Though weakness is progressive, it nevertheless often shows periods of *apparent* arrest. This slowing is often most obvious either in the very early stages or, more often, when a person first starts needing a wheelchair. At present we know of no way of completely arresting the course of the disease, but with physiotherapy and other measures it is possible to prevent or delay certain complications, such as *contractures*. These are usually the result of prolonged immobilization, when joints can become fixed and can no longer be moved freely.

The course and severity of a disease, its *prognosis*, depend very much on the particular type of dystrophy from which a person suffers. A precise diagnosis is therefore essential. This is possible from a careful examination by a doctor experienced in the disease and by relevant laboratory tests. Features of the various types of dystrophy will be discussed in more detail in Chapter 4.

Weakness is *not* usually associated with pain and the muscles are not tender to touch. There are usually few complaints apart from those that result from weakness of the affected muscles. Sometimes, especially in those types of dystrophy that mainly affect the major limb muscles, cramps and stiffness are quite common. However, *severe* cramps and stiffness are very unusual and, especially if the muscles are also tender, may indicate some other cause for the muscle weakness.

Sometimes in certain types of dystrophy, some muscles actually seem to be enlarged rather than wasted. In athletes muscle enlargement is, of course, common. In dystrophy, however, the enlarged muscles are weak, and their enlargement has therefore been referred to as *pseudohypertrophy* (which means false hypertrophy). The calf muscles are most often affected in this way but other muscles may also become similarly enlarged. The cause of pseudohypertrophy is not entirely clear but is probably largely due to the muscle tissue becoming replaced by fat. Duchenne muscular dystrophy, in which this is a prominent feature, was often referred to in the past as 'pseudohypertrophic muscular dystrophy'. However, pseudohypertrophy can occur in several other different types of dystrophy as well.

Types of muscle

So far we have been considering muscle as merely the tissue responsible for moving limbs. The thigh muscles straighten and extend the knee, for example, and the shoulder muscles raise the arms. These are referred to as *voluntary* muscles because they are under voluntary control. You can will your arm to be raised and the message from your brain descends through the spinal cord to exit at the appropriate point via the nerves supplying the relevant muscles. As these muscles mainly, but not exclusively, move bones that are hinged at joints, they are often also referred to as *skeletal* muscles. The muscles of respiration are somewhat of an exception because you can partly control their function, by holding your breath, but usually you are unaware of their activity.

There are no less than 434 different voluntary muscles in the human body, and one of the banes of the medical student's life is knowing the positions and functions of all these muscles! In an adult they constitute over 40 per cent of the total body weight. This explains why weight loss is not uncommon in patients with any degree of muscle wasting, though to some extent this can be compensated for by energy conservation resulting from lack of physical activity. In fact, in some individuals, when physical activity becomes severely restricted, weight gain becomes a serious problem, and the only remedy is restriction of calorie intake by dieting.

Apart from voluntary muscle, there are two other types of muscle (heart and smooth) that are referred to as being *involuntary* because neither of them is under voluntary control. Though some people believe they can, for a period, slow their heart rate, most of us are unable to control this important function. Similarly, the smooth muscle that surrounds the wall of the intestines and is responsible for involuntary contractions that propel the contents along (called peristalsis) cannot be controlled voluntarily. In some dystrophies heart muscle and smooth muscle may become involved. For example, when the heart is affected this can result in breathlessness at rest. However, only in certain types of dystrophy is this a predominant feature. Involvement of the smooth muscle of the gut may account, at least in part, for constipation, though this is more likely to be due to reduced physical activity and lack of dietary fibre.

Muscle structure

Muscles are composed of bundles of muscle fibres, and it is these bundles that are visible to the naked eye when a joint of meat is cut across (Fig. 2.2). The bundles form the bulk of each muscle, except at either end where the tendons are located. With some exceptions, such as the eye muscles, each tendon attaches a muscle to bones on either side of a joint. When the muscle contracts the relevant joint therefore bends (flexes) or straightens (extends).

The important element of muscle tissue is the *muscle fibre*. Each fibre is formed from several individual muscle cells that fuse together during fetal development so that each mature muscle fibre comes to contain several nuclei. Individual muscle fibres vary in length from one muscle to another. In the small muscles of the eye, for example, they are only a few millimetres long, but they are up to several centimetres long in the large muscles of the limbs.

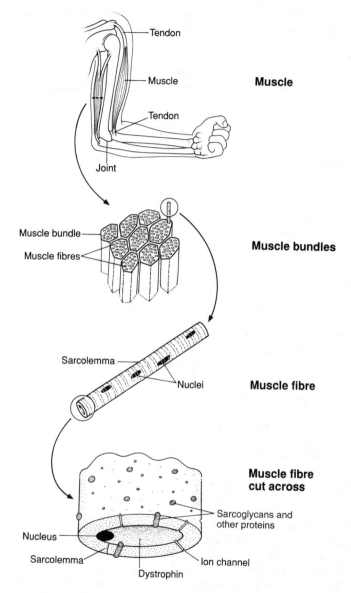

Figure 2.2 Diagram of the relationship between muscle, muscle bundles, muscle fibres, and the muscle fibre membrane (sarcolemma).

Each muscle fibre is enclosed in a skin or membrane called the *sarcolemma*. This covering of each muscle fibre is a complicated structure. Studies with powerful electron microscopes have shown that it consists of two layers. Traversing between these two layers are minute pores or channels that open and close and that allow certain *ions* (electrically charged atoms such as sodium and calcium) to pass backwards and forwards across the membrane. The free movement of these ions is an important process in muscle contraction.

On the inner side of the two layers is a lattice-like arrangement of protein molecules that holds the membrane together and stops it from tearing when the muscle contracts. An important protein in the lattice structure is *dystrophin*. It was discovered in 1987 that this protein is absent in Duchenne muscular dystrophy, and this led to our present understanding of the disease. The word dystrophin was, of course, derived from dystrophy, so emphasizing its importance in the disease—though at the time it was discovered some argued that the word was really not appropriate as dystrophin was only present in normal muscle. However, it is now universally accepted for the name of the protein that is absent in Duchenne muscular dystrophy.

Cause of muscle weakness

In Duchenne muscular dystrophy, dystrophin is absent because the responsible gene fails to make this protein. In the clinically similar, but much milder, disorder of Becker muscular dystrophy, the responsible gene synthesizes dystrophin but the protein is abnormal. Dystrophin, along with other related proteins to which it is attached and anchored to the membrane, is responsible for retaining the structure of the muscle fibre membrane. If dystrophin is defective then the membrane breaks down and becomes 'leaky'. That is, substances and molecules within the fibre leak out into the circulation. Among the substances that leak out is a muscle enzyme called *creatine kinase*. Enzymes are proteins within the cell that are necessary for certain chemical reactions and creatine kinase is necessary for producing energy for muscle contraction. In several types of dystrophy, most notably Duchenne and Becker dystrophies, the level of this enzyme in the blood is far higher than in normal people. The measurement of the level of this enzyme in a blood sample therefore provides a very useful test for these diseases.

In the last few years the basic underlying protein defects in many other forms of dystrophy have been identified. Most of these proteins are located on the inside of the sarcolemma, such as dystrophin, within the sarcolemma itself, or even on the surface of the muscle fibre (Fig. 2.3). Those proteins defective in particular forms of dystrophy include, for example, laminin α2 (also known

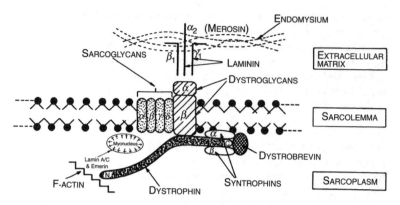

Figure 2.3 Diagram of the various proteins associated with the muscle sarcolemma or muscle nucleus (myonucleus).

as merosin), caveolin, various sarcoglycans, dysferlin, and dystrophin. The absence of any one of these proteins results in the disruption and breakdown of the muscle membrane and is probably the explanation for the weakness in these disorders. However, there are two exceptions referred to as lamin A/C and emerin proteins. These proteins are not associated with the sarcolemma but are located on the inner surface of the muscle nuclei (myonuclei)! How a deficiency of these proteins results in weakness is at present a complete mystery.

Many scientists believe that weakness is partly due to a leak of substances *from* the muscle fibre, which are essential for muscle contraction. But it may also be due to substances leaking *into* the fibre that then damage processes necessary for muscle contraction and perhaps at the same time cause irreparable damage to the fibre. Calcium may be important in this way because it is well known that an increase in the level of calcium in cells results in damage to biochemical processes, which are essential for cell survival. Knowledge of the trail of events that ultimately results in muscle cell damage and muscle weakness can lead to rational approaches to possible treatment.

Animal studies of dystrophy

For obvious reasons it is very rarely possible to study different tissues from any one affected person. And of course for ethical reasons it is difficult to test experimental treatments that might prove to have untoward and serious side-effects. For these reasons, some scientists have turned their attention to animal studies. In the past, various strains of animals with muscle weakness have been studied in this way, including mink, sheep, duck, cow, and chicken.

But none of these has proved to be strictly comparable with human muscular dystrophy. However, more recently two 'animal models' have been found with diseases that are genetically and biochemically very similar to the human condition. These are the so-called *mdx* dystrophic mouse and a particular strain of golden retriever dog. Of these, the latter is proving the best model of Duchenne dystrophy, and could prove an excellent subject for studying the effects and value of any new treatments.

Some unanswered questions

Though the picture has become very much clearer in the last few years, there are still many questions about muscular dystrophy that remain unanswered. For example, though we now know that a deficiency of dystrophin is the basic cause of Duchenne muscular dystrophy, we still have no idea why the disease only becomes obvious around school age when we know that the defect is present even before birth. This is also true of Becker muscular dystrophy, yet here the disease may not become obvious until the twenties or even thirties. In the *mdx* mouse model there is the same absence of dystrophin but the mouse does not become progressively weaker or die from the disease. Why in the human disease are some muscles (for example, those of the limbs) more affected than others? The facial muscles, for example, are rarely severely affected, except in one particular type of dystrophy (facioscapulohumeral muscular dystrophy), and chewing and swallowing are never affected (apart from in oculopharyngeal muscular dystrophy), nor are bladder and bowel control affected. Furthermore, as we have discussed already, why do some people with dystrophy become more severely affected than relatives of the same age with the same disorder? Answers to these and related problems will no doubt be found with further research in the next few years. Until then, we have to accept that there are many questions to which we still do not have answers.

3

Confirming the diagnosis

> **Key points**
>
> ◆ Most essential in the diagnosis of muscular dystrophy is a careful clinical examination by an experienced doctor.
>
> ◆ In order to confirm a case of dystrophy a blood test (for serum creatine kinase levels and in rare forms resort may have to be made to DNA studies as well), electromyography, and muscle biopsy are important.
>
> ◆ By using certain tests (DNA and special muscle protein stains) it is now possible in most cases to make the diagnosis of a specific type of dystrophy, which is important in order to assess the possible course of the disease in a person and for reliable genetic counselling.

It has been said that an experienced and astute physician can often make the diagnosis of muscular dystrophy without resort to any laboratory tests. In a family in which others have already been diagnosed as having the disease, this is probably true. For example, if a boy has been diagnosed as having Duchenne muscular dystrophy and now his younger brother is found to have enlarged calves and difficulty in running and climbing stairs, then it seems more than likely that he too is becoming afflicted with the same disease. However, the situation is not always so straightforward. A patient's impressions about his or her relatives who have not been examined can be misleading.

This is a notorious problem, for example, in facioscapulohumeral muscular dystrophy. Here relatives are sometimes described as being unaffected when they are in fact in the early stages of the disease: facial appearance may be misinterpreted as familial likeness rather than as an expression of facial weakness, and early weakness of the shoulder muscles may go unrecognized by both the patient and his or her relatives.

Not only may details given by relatives be misleading, but even a careful clinical examination may not always provide all the answers. For example, an early sign of weakness of the hip muscles is a so-called *waddling gait*; that is, the individual sways from side to side when walking. This is very common in various types of muscular dystrophy when the hip muscles are affected. But as a famous paediatrician has emphasized 'not everyone who waddles has muscular dystrophy'. Any disease that causes hip weakness will result in a waddling gait.

An important reason for confirming a suspected diagnosis of dystrophy with further tests, particularly in children, was to exclude the possibility of polymyositis, which can closely mimic the disease. Thankfully, the disease is now very rare in Western countries.

Finally, and most importantly, the diagnosis of muscular dystrophy, and particularly the *type* of dystrophy, is essential for two reasons: first in order to be able to assess the possible course of the disease, which is important for future planning, and secondly to determine the mode of inheritance, which is essential for genetic counselling.

Therefore, though the doctor may be fairly convinced of the diagnosis after taking a detailed medical history and a careful physical examination, further tests are invariably necessary in order to confirm the diagnosis of what is after all a serious disease.

There are essentially three diagnostic tests that are often used in this way: a blood test, electromyography, and a muscle biopsy.

Blood tests

Two blood tests are used in the diagnosis of dystrophy: one is to measure the level of the enzyme *creatine kinase* in a test tube, and the other is for *DNA studies*. It is possible to do both tests on the same sample of blood and at the same time, though often DNA studies may be delayed until a later date.

The CPK test

As we have seen (Chapter 2), creatine kinase (CK), often called creatine phosphokinase (CPK), is an important muscle enzyme which in several types of dystrophy leaks into the circulation from the muscle, an observation first made over 50 years ago by Setsuro Ebashi in Japan and Jean-Claude Dreyfus in Paris. In normal healthy people the level ranges from about 100 to 200 units, being slightly higher in males than in females. Levels are somewhat raised (200–300 units) in normal newborn babies and in normal children and adults after vigorous exercise. In comparison, the levels in Duchenne muscular dystrophy, even in newborn baby boys, are grossly elevated (50–100 times normal). This also occurs in the early stages of Becker muscular dystrophy. Such grossly elevated levels occur in very few other conditions in children, and these can be excluded on the medical history and physical examination. Thus a young boy who is having increasing difficulty running, rising from a chair, or climbing stairs, who has enlarged calves, and is found to have a *grossly* elevated CK level is almost certain to have Duchenne muscular dystrophy. In an adult suspected of having Becker muscular dystrophy the situation is a little more complicated because in adulthood there are several conditions that can result in similarly raised CK levels, but these can usually be excluded on the basis of the medical history and results of the physical examination.

Moderately elevated levels (up to 10 times normal) can occur in some other forms of muscular dystrophy (notably limb girdle, Emery–Dreifuss, and facioscapulohumeral muscular dystrophies) and here the test is less helpful in establishing a diagnosis because there can be many causes for such levels of CK. Finally, slight elevations (up to about five times normal) can occur in healthy females who carry the gene for Duchenne and Becker muscular dystrophies. Therefore, with certain reservations (to be discussed later; Chapter 8), this can be a useful test in helping to identify such carriers.

The CK test is simple to perform, requiring at most a *venepuncture* where a small sample of blood is removed from a vein, usually at the elbow, or in small children by a heel prick. Its further attraction is that it is very inexpensive to carry out! This is an extremely useful test in diagnosis but its limitations have to be recognized. It is not a specific test for dystrophy.

DNA studies

For genetic studies a blood sample is usually also required. In this case it is not the level of a chemical in the blood serum that is studied, but DNA and gene markers in the white cells (leucocytes). As far as the patient is concerned, this involves no more than for a CPK test—that is, a small sample of blood is removed from a vein at the elbow by venepuncture—but the laboratory studies themselves are much more complicated and require considerable expertise.

DNA studies involve first separating off the leucocytes from the blood sample and then extracting DNA from these cells. The DNA is then examined by various molecular genetic techniques. The most widely used is called *Southern blot* after Ed Southern who invented and developed the technique. It will tell us if a specific mutant gene is present or absent. If the mutant gene that causes a particular type of dystrophy is known, as in the case of Duchenne and Becker muscular dystrophies, these DNA tests can tell us whether or not the mutant gene is present in a particular patient. If the mutant gene is present, then the diagnosis of a specific type of dystrophy can be made with confidence.

Mutations in particular genes have now been identified for most forms of dystrophy. Unfortunately, for a few types of dystrophy the genes involved have not yet been identified, although their chromosomal locations are known. In this case DNA tests are carried out not only on the affected person but also on relatives in order to determine if the disease is inherited along with an identifiable DNA marker which is known to be very close to the mutant gene on a particular chromosome. If a person proves to have the marker, then he or she may therefore possess the disease gene as well. These latter studies are complex and time-consuming. Fortunately, they will become less necessary as we are able to identify the specific mutant gene in each type of dystrophy. Details of these DNA studies can be found in several modern texts listed at the end of the book.

Electromyography

When muscles contract, they generate small amounts of electricity. This electrical activity can be detected by inserting a small needle (called an *electrode*) into the muscle and amplifying the small amount of electrical activity produced. This activity can then be displayed on an oscilloscope, a sort of TV screen. This technique of recording electrical activity from contracting muscle fibres is referred to as electromyography or EMG. The electrical activity appears as a blip or wave on the screen, which is known as an *action potential.*

The study of the shape and size of these action potentials provides very useful information about the muscle and is a very valuable diagnostic aid in neuromuscular disorders. For example, in the muscular dystrophies the action potentials are very small, whereas in other diseases they may be very large (so-called 'giant potentials'). Furthermore, in healthy individuals, as well as in those with dystrophy, after an electrode has been inserted into the muscle there are no potentials when the muscle is at rest. On the other hand, in certain other disorders (such as spinal muscular atrophy and Lou Gehrig's disease or amyotrophic lateral sclerosis) there are spontaneous bursts of small potentials. Thus an EMG examination can be used to confirm the diagnosis of dystrophy and distinguish this from other types of neuromuscular disease, but it cannot tell us what type of dystrophy a patient may have.

Unfortunately an EMG does involve having a needle-electrode inserted into a muscle (sometimes into several muscles) and not everyone is able to tolerate this, though actually it causes no more discomfort than a pin prick. It is, however, a difficult test to perform in small children as the patient's cooperation, in voluntarily contracting various muscle groups, is important. For these reasons the test is becoming less widely used in diagnosing muscular dystrophy, especially in children. It is perhaps more important in diagnosing non-dystrophic muscle diseases, especially in adults.

Muscle biopsy

After the CPK test, the most important method for diagnosing dystrophy is a muscle biopsy.

The technique involves removing a small amount of tissue from a muscle that is clearly affected, but not severely so. If a severely affected muscle is biopsied, then the material obtained may contain mainly fat with little actual muscle tissue on which the diagnosis can be made.

There are two ways in which a muscle biopsy may be performed: an *open* biopsy or a *needle* biopsy.

An open biopsy

An open biopsy, as the name implies, involves making a small cut in the skin (about 2–3 cm) and then removing a piece of the underlying muscle under sterile operative conditions. This can be done with local anaesthesia though most prefer a general anaesthetic so that they can be unaware of the surgeon's activities.

A needle biopsy

This involves inserting a sterile, special cutting, and hollow biopsy needle under local anaesthetic through the skin and into the muscle. A small fragment of muscle is then sucked up the needle and withdrawn.

However, all surgical operations that involve general anaesthesia, no matter how minor (and a muscle biopsy is considered a minor surgical operation), involve some risk. In patients with dystrophy the risk can be greater than normal. Patients do not always tolerate anaesthetic agents well and, in any event, their lung and heart functions may already be somewhat compromised by the disease (see Chapter 5). For these reasons needle biopsy is gaining favour. Although Duchenne himself, the French neurologist after whom the disease Duchenne muscular dystrophy is named, advocated the use of the biopsy needle over 100 years ago, for a long time this did not meet with much support. This was largely because it was seen as a 'blind' procedure and therefore there might be the danger of inadvertently damaging nerves or blood vessels. In fact, with modern equipment, such hazards are very rare and for this reason many doctors now prefer to use this technique as it does not require general anaesthesia. Some medical scientists in their research have even been known to carry out the procedure repeatedly on themselves with no untoward effects.

Muscle histology

Once a small piece of muscle has been removed, it is taken to the laboratory and after careful preparation thin sections are cut. These sections are placed on a glass slide and stained, and then carefully examined under the microscope. The microscopic study of tissues in this way is referred to as *histology*. In a clear-cut case the difference in appearance from normal muscle is quite striking (Fig. 3.1). Normally, muscle fibres are of fairly uniform size and packed closely together with little fatty or fibrous tissue between them. However, in dystrophy the muscle fibres vary greatly in diameter—some are very large and others very small. Furthermore, many of the fibres often appear to be breaking down (*necrosis*) and being invaded by certain other cells called *macrophages*, which consume them (phagocytosis). Ultimately, almost all the muscle fibres may be destroyed in this way and replaced by fatty–fibrous tissue.

In less severe types of dystrophy, and in minimally affected muscles from severe cases, not all these changes may be very evident. The pathologist's skill then comes into play in interpreting minimal changes that indicate dystrophy.

Muscle histochemistry

The various changes described above can occur in almost all types of dystrophy and are not specific to any particular type. An important recent development in this regard, however, has been the use of stains that identify specific proteins known to be abnormal in some way in particular types of dystrophy. The microscopic study of tissues using chemical stains in this way is referred

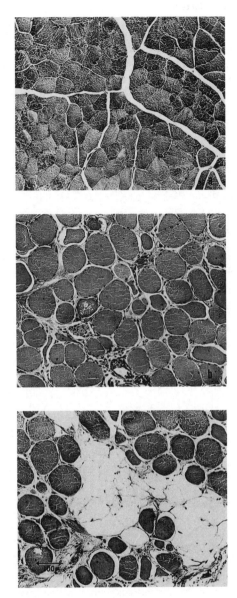

Figure 3.1 Muscle histology. *Top*: normal muscle fibres are uniform in size; *middle*: early Duchenne dystrophy with variation in fibre size with occasional fibres undergoing necrosis and phagocytosis; *bottom*: late dystrophy with many fibres replaced by fatty–fibrous tissue.

to as *histochemistry*. For example, chemical stains are now available for identifying dystrophin. In normal tissue the outer membrane (sarcolemma) of all the muscle fibres stains uniformly for dystrophin. In Duchenne muscular dystrophy, where dystrophin is absent, the muscle fibres fail to stain at all. In Becker muscular dystrophy, where dystrophin is present but abnormal, most fibres do stain but the staining is not uniform and varies a great deal from one fibre to another. This variability with dystrophin stains gives a clue to the diagnosis.

Histochemical tests are now available to identify the specific protein abnormalities in almost all dystrophies (Chapter 2), and therefore can be used to establish a precise diagnosis.

Other investigations

Apart from a blood test, EMG, and muscle biopsy, other tests may also be requested by the physician, depending on a particular person's problems. For example, an electrocardiogram (ECG or EKG) is essential to check the heart. This, or echocardiography, is a simple straightforward painless investigation to allow the activity of the heart to be recorded and studied. Ultrasound and computerized tomography (CT *scan*), and more recently magnetic resonance imaging (MRI scan), are sometimes also used nowadays to show up and localize muscle weakness. These tests are non-invasive and painless procedures.

4

Different types of muscular dystrophy

⮕ Key points

◆ There are many different types of muscular dystrophy depending on distribution of predominantly affected muscle groups (Fig. 4.1), severity and prognosis, modes of inheritance, and genetic defects.

◆ It is possible on the basis of the distribution of predominant muscle wasting and weakness, along with certain other features, such as age at onset, to define at least eight *major* types of muscular dystrophy. Myotonic dystrophy is unique in so many ways that it should perhaps not really be considered a muscular dystrophy; it has been included here for completeness.

◆ A precise diagnosis of a specific type of dystrophy (based on muscle histochemistry and DNA studies) is essential in order to determine the probable course and outcome of the disease in an affected person and for reliable genetic counselling.

The muscular dystrophies have been defined as a group of genetic disorders with progressive muscle wasting and weakness where the disease primarily involves muscle in which there are characteristic microscopic changes (see Chapter 3). However, as we have mentioned, muscular dystrophy is not one disease. In fact over 30 different types have so far been recognized. Some of these, however, are very rare or occur only in certain parts of the world. The existence of others is a matter of debate, but as we learn more of the causes of these various conditions much of this confusion will no doubt be resolved. Here we shall limit our discussion to those main types of dystrophy that are well defined and relatively frequent.

These various types are diagnosed on the basis of the distribution of the groups of muscles that are *predominantly* affected (Fig. 4.1).

In the very early stages of dystrophy, when weakness is first noticed, often only one group of muscles may be affected. On the other hand, late in the course

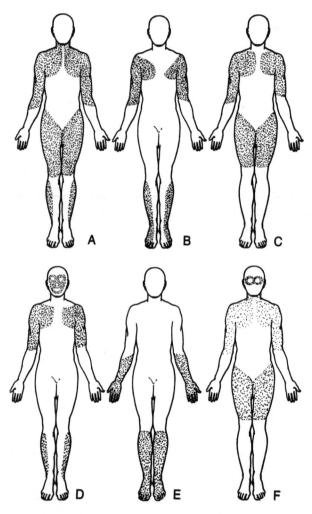

Figure 4.1 Distribution of predominantly affected muscle groups in various dystrophies. **A** Duchenne and Becker; **B** Emery–Dreifuss; **C** limb gridle; **D** facioscapulohumeral; **E** distal; **F** oculopharyngeal.

of the disease, weakness may become so widespread as to blur its distribution, which at first was distinctive and characterized a particular type of dystrophy. For these reasons in the very early, as well as the late, stages of dystrophy it may sometimes be difficult to make a diagnosis of a specific type.

Bearing this in mind it is nevertheless possible in many cases to decide on a type of dystrophy from the distribution of predominant muscle weakness as well as from various other features. The main types are:

◆ Duchenne muscular dystrophy

◆ Becker muscular dystrophy

◆ Emery–Dreifuss muscular dystrophy

◆ limb girdle muscular dystrophy

◆ facioscapulohumeral muscular dystrophy

◆ distal muscular dystrophy

◆ oculopharyngeal muscular dystrophy

◆ congenital muscular dystrophy.

For completeness *myotonic dystrophy* will also be discussed, though this is unique in so many different ways that some no longer consider it a muscular dystrophy.

Duchenne muscular dystrophy

This, the commonest form of dystrophy, is named after the French neurologist Guillaume Benjamin Amand Duchenne (Fig. 4.2), or Duchenne de Boulogne (1806–1875), who described the disease in his book *De l'electrisation localisée* of 1861 and in greater detail in several publications in 1868. However, as so often happens in the history of medicine, there is some disagreement as to who actually described the disease first. In fact recent historical research has now revealed that the English physician Edward Meryon (1807–1880) (Fig. 4.3) described the disease in considerable detail several years before Duchenne and quite independently. However, the appellation Duchenne muscular dystrophy is so well established that it would be a brave person who now tried to change it.

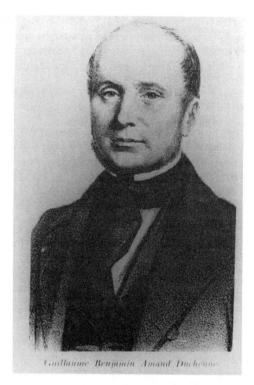

Guillaume Benjamin Amand Duchenne

Figure 4.2 Duchenne de Boulogne (1806–1875). (Reproduced from *The founders of neurology*, edited by Webb Haymaker, 1953. Courtesy of Charles C. Thomas, Publishers, Springfield, Illinois.)

Duchenne muscular dystrophy is due to a mutation on the X chromosome and is therefore inherited as a so-called X-linked trait. This will be discussed further in Chapter 8. It means, however, that only boys are usually affected.

The onset is often ill-defined. Looking back over the child's history, there may have been some delay in learning to walk. In one survey of affected boys about half had not been walking by the age of 18 months, whereas almost all normal children are walking by this age. Sometimes the first thing parents notice is that the calf muscles are enlarged, but usually medical attention is not sought until the parents begin to realize that something seems to be seriously wrong. They may become aware that their son falls over more than other children, or he is never able to run well, or cannot get up from the floor or climb

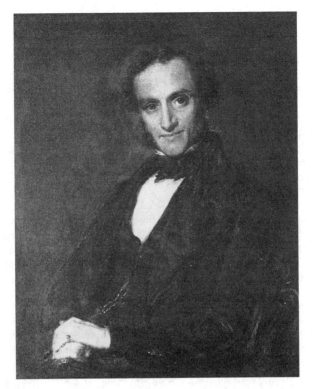

Figure 4.3 Edward Meryon (1807–1880). (By John Linnell, private collection).

stairs properly. It has been said that any little boy who shows signs of a problem with muscle development should have a creatine phosphokinase test to exclude the possibility of Duchenne muscular dystrophy.

Sometimes the diagnosis of Duchenne muscular dystrophy is not made until school age. By then difficulty in walking is usually obvious. He often walks:

- on his toes

- with his abdomen pushed forwards

- with a waddling gait.

These are early hallmarks of the disease and result from weakness of muscles of the pelvis, which normally extend the hips in order to retain the upright

27

position when standing. When these muscles are weak there is a tendency for the pelvis to tilt forward, and in order to compensate for this the affected boy pushes his abdomen forward and his shoulders backward. This results in what is called *lordosis* as it resembles the gait of a peer of the realm.

Rising from the floor unaided also becomes increasingly difficult, which, like the waddling gait, is due to weakness of the muscles around the hips. This results in what is referred to as *Gower's sign* after the English physician who first described it. Whenever there is weakness of the hip muscles (which is not limited to Duchenne muscular dystrophy but can also occur in other dystrophies and diseases) when attempting to rise, the person presses on his thighs and then climbs up them in order to extend the hips and straighten up (Fig. 4.4).

At the same time that weakness of the hip muscles becomes evident, there is also weakness of the shoulder muscles so that the affected boy has increasing difficulty raising his arms. The hip and shoulder muscles are referred to as *proximal* muscles, as opposed to *distal* muscles of the lower legs and forearms. The weakness, at least at the beginning, is therefore mainly proximal in this disease.

As weakness of the hips and thighs progresses, so walking becomes increasingly difficult and affected boys usually become confined to a wheelchair by the age of 12. Thereafter the rate of progression of the disease usually becomes less obvious. Most muscle groups later become affected. However, the eye muscles are always spared and chewing and swallowing are unaffected. When confined to a wheelchair the problem is that such immobility increases the likelihood of *contractures* developing (Chapter 5). The sole of the foot often turns inwards, which is referred to as *talipes*. Flexion contractures of the knees and elbows later develop so that the legs and arms can no longer be straightened out. But much more seriously, with prolonged sitting in one position the spine gradually curves to one side and so compresses the lung on that side. This is referred to as *scoliosis* and can result in serious problems with breathing and chest infections. One of the main challenges in the treatment of those with dystrophy who become confined to a wheelchair is to prevent this from happening. This can be achieved to some extent by always adopting an upright sitting position and the use of a back support, but perhaps more effectively by surgery (see Chapter 5). In fact respiratory problems are the main cause of death in these boys, which usually occurs in the late teens or early twenties without adequate treatment. We know that the heart is also affected in the disease and this may aggravate any respiratory problems, but does not usually in itself give cause for special treatment.

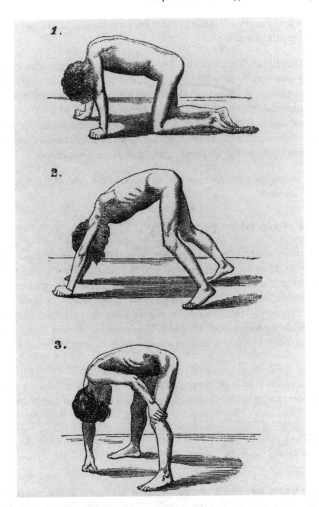

Figure 4.4 Gower's sign or manoeuvre from his book *Pseudohypertrophic muscular paralysis* published in 1879.

Apart from muscle weakness, affected boys often have very few health problems. It is now clear, however, that up to a third of boys with Duchenne muscular dystrophy have some degree of intellectual impairment. This is particularly reflected in poor reading ability, word comprehension, and memory skills. This intellectual impairment is *not* related to muscle weakness and is *not* progressive. A small proportion (less than 1 in 20) have a severe degree of mental handicap.

It seems that the depression of intellect, like the muscle weakness, is due to a deficiency of the protein dystrophin, but in this case it is dystrophin located in the brain cells that is abnormal. This deficiency of brain dystrophin somehow results in mental impairment. But how this occurs and why only some boys are affected and not others is ill understood at the present time. Many affected boys have no impairment of intellect and I personally know of several who have reached college and university standards in their education.

Epilepsy is not particularly frequent in this disease, and visual and hearing acuity are normal.

Becker muscular dystrophy

This form of dystrophy is so named after the late Peter Emil Becker, Professor of Human Genetics at the University of Göttingen, who first described the disorder and clearly distinguished it from other dystrophies in the mid-1950s. It is caused by mutations of the gene that also causes Duchenne muscular dystrophy. In this case the mutant gene does synthesize dystrophin but the protein produced is abnormal. This explains why, in many ways, the disease so much resembles Duchenne muscular dystrophy but is much less severe.

As in Duchenne muscular dystrophy, weakness mainly affects the proximal limb muscles and pseudohypertrophy of the calf muscles is also common.

Onset is usually in the teens or early twenties, with toe walking, a wad-dling gait, and the development of lordosis.

Although weakness almost always begins in the lower limbs, eventually the upper limb musculature also becomes involved. Affected men usually become confined to a wheelchair in their thirties, but this is quite variable. Some never require a wheelchair and cope with everyday living using various aids. Once confined to a wheelchair, however, all the problems attendant on immobiliza-tion can occur, as in Duchenne muscular dystrophy. In some cases cardiac involvement may be the predominant feature. In any event, all individuals with Becker dystrophy should be periodically seen by a cardiologist for evidence of heart disease, which can be treated. Some degree of intellectual impairment may occur in this disease but it is less common than in Duchenne muscular dystrophy.

Death may occur in the twenties or thirties but often affected men survive into middle age and beyond. Because affected males survive into adulthood, not infrequently they marry and have children. As we shall see (Chapter 8) all their sons will be normal, but all their daughters will be carriers who are therefore at risk of having affected sons. Thus families with a number of affected individuals are not uncommon with this condition.

Becker muscular dystrophy was at one time considered to be rare. However, recent DNA studies in affected males with no family history of the disease, who were thought previously to have other disorders, have now shown many of them to have Becker muscular dystrophy. The result is that we now believe that although it is rarer than Duchenne muscular dystrophy, it is probably commoner than many other dystrophies.

Different mutations of the Duchenne gene are now known to result in a spectrum of diseases. At one extreme there is the severe Duchenne type of muscular dystrophy, followed by boys with relatively early onset but who survive longer than in classical Duchenne dystrophy, males with Becker muscular dystrophy, and finally, at the other extreme, men who develop relatively mild weakness only in later life. Such a spectrum reflects different mutations of this gene and their different effects on the synthesis of dystrophin. Detailed knowledge of the mutation and its effect on dystrophin synthesis provide the best ways for determining the precise diagnosis and ultimate course of the disease in a particular person.

Emery–Dreifuss muscular dystrophy

This is an uncommon type of dystrophy, but because it is so distinctive and because early recognition and appropriate treatment can be life saving, it deserves special mention. Cases of this disease have no doubt been noted by physicians in the past, but it was described in detail for the first time in the mid-1960s by Fritz Dreifuss of Charlottesville, USA, and myself. The recognition of this type of dystrophy grew out of studies of a large family in Virginia, USA, with the disease which did not fit into any of the types of dystrophy that had been described up to that time. We therefore considered it a separate disease. This has since been confirmed by others, and individuals and families with this disease have now been reported from various parts of the world.

It is a relatively benign muscular dystrophy which, like Becker muscular dystrophy, can be inherited as an X-linked recessive trait in some families.

However, in other families the disorder is inherited as an autosomal dominant or, very rarely, autosomal recessive trait. Apart from the latter, which has only been reported in very severely affected young children, in all other much commoner X-linked or autosomal dominant cases weakness predominantly affects the shoulder and upper arm muscles as well as the anterior tibial and peroneal muscles of the lower legs (Fig. 4.1). The latter raise the foot and so the main complaint at the beginning is not so much difficulty in climbing stairs, for example, but a tendency to trip over carpets and steps. Later on, the pelvic girdle musculature also becomes affected and some people require a wheelchair in later life.

Apart from this distinctive distribution of muscle weakness, another distinguishing feature is the *early* development of muscle contractures *before* there is any significant degree of muscle weakness. These contractures predominantly affect three regions of the body:

◆ the heel cords (Achilles tendons)—so from an early age affected boys walk on their toes

◆ elbows—so that the elbows cannot be extended fully even from childhood

◆ muscles at the back of the neck—so that bending the neck forward is difficult.

There is never any calf enlargement or pseudohypertrophy. The progression is relatively slow and most affected individuals survive into middle age with varying degrees of incapacity. There does not appear to be any intellectual impairment, but there is one other feature that is singularly important.

The heart often becomes affected in a very distinctive way, which is referred to as *heart block* and results in abnormal slowing of the heart rate. This does not occur in every patient and may not develop until later in life. On the other hand, exceptionally it may occur in youth before significant weakness is apparent. It has to be recognized because effective treatment (which often involves inserting a pacemaker or even a defibrillator) is life saving (individuals with a pacemaker can then live more or less normal lives). One man I know with this condition who has a pacemaker is a keen naturalist and has crossed the Sahara in quest of specimens, though such feats are not recommended for most patients.

Features which indicate that heart block may be developing include:

◆ slowing of the pulse rate

◆ drowsiness

◆ dizzy spells

◆ fainting attacks.

If these symptoms develop in a man with this condition, medical advice should be sought immediately. In any event, all individuals with this disorder should be seen regularly by a cardiologist.

Limb girdle muscular dystrophy

In this type of dystrophy weakness predominantly affects the *limb girdle* muscles, that is, the muscles around the hips and shoulders. However, there are many causes for such limb girdle weakness. They include, for example:

◆ certain rare congenital myopathies

◆ spinal muscular atrophies

◆ polymyositis

◆ so-called acquired myopathies associated with various glandular disturbances.

Even certain infections and some drugs, most notably steroids, may produce limb girdle weakness. These possibilities have to be excluded by a careful medical examination and by appropriate tests.

Limb girdle weakness in a female may be due to her being a so-called *manifesting carrier* of Duchenne muscular dystrophy. This is not common but has to be considered because such a woman is at risk of having sons affected with the disease (see Chapter 8). Also limb girdle weakness in a male may be due to Becker *muscular dystrophy* and this can also be a diagnostic problem when no one else in the family is affected. Thankfully both these latter possibilities can now be excluded by appropriate DNA and muscle dystrophin studies (see Chapter 3). If these two possibilities are excluded, we are left with a group of disorders that we refer to as the limb girdle muscular dystrophies, as there are now recognized to be several types of this disease. They differ in their age at onset, severity, and mode of inheritance.

In all cases there is involvement of the shoulder girdle and hip girdle muscu-lature. The weakness may be progressive and can eventually extend to other muscles. A wheelchair may become necessary after several years and contrac-tures and scoliosis may then develop. Thereafter respiratory function often declines and life expectancy is reduced. However, the disease is quite variable. In some it is very slowly progressive and affected people can remain mobile throughout their lives. Intellect is unimpaired.

Recent studies have shown that limb girdle dystrophy can be divided into two main groups, which are inherited differently and differ in severity. First, there are autosomal dominant forms where the disease affects both sexes and is transmitted from one generation to another (see Chapter 8). So far seven dif-ferent types of dominant limb girdle dystrophy have been described. Generally onset is after childhood and they tend to be mild in severity though in some cases the heart may be affected. Secondly, 13 different autosomal recessive forms of the disease have so far been described. Here the disorder only affects siblings, parents being perfectly healthy (Chapter 8). Onset is in childhood and tends to be more severe than the dominant forms. The genes for all these recessive forms have now been located and several forms have been shown to be due to defects of various sarcoglycans or dysferlin (Chapter 2). One form is due to a deficiency of a muscle enzyme known as calpain-3. In many cases the autosomal recessive forms resemble Duchenne dystrophy but here girls may also be affected. The distinction from Duchenne dystrophy and a specific diagnosis is made on the basis of histochemical and biochemical studies on muscle biopsy material (Chapter 3).

The distinction from Duchenne muscular dystrophy is particularly important because, though the outcome may be very similar, the mode of inheritance is quite different. In Duchenne muscular dystrophy a healthy sister may prove to be a carrier and therefore at high risk of having affected sons. In this dis-order, because it is inherited as an autosomal recessive trait, an unaffected sister is most unlikely to have affected children. This is a rare disorder in North America and western Europe where it is roughly 20 times less common than the clinically similar Duchenne type of dystrophy. It seems to be more common in Brazil and certain Arab communities, most notably in northern Africa.

Facioscapulohumeral muscular dystrophy

As the name implies there is facial weakness that results in an inability to close the eyes properly and to whistle. The smile is often described as being 'transverse' and the lips appear to pout. Speech may become indistinct if the facial weakness is marked. The other characteristic feature is wasting and weakness of the shoulder muscles, particularly around the shoulder blades or scapulae. The shoulders droop and there is increasing difficulty in raising the arms. A notable feature is that the shoulder blades become very prominent, for which the term 'winging' is often used. This disorder is an exception to the general rule that in dystrophy weakness is usually symmetrical: in facioscapulohumeral muscular dystrophy, muscle weakness often affects one side more than the other at the beginning.

The other muscles affected early on are the anterior tibial and peroneal muscles, which raise the foot, so that tripping over carpets and steps is a frequent problem; there is a 'stepping gait' and running becomes impossible.

As the disease progresses the pelvic girdle musculature may also become affected with a resultant waddling gait and lordosis, and people affected in this way may eventually require a wheelchair. Hearing loss, which may be unilateral, is not infrequent. This is now recognized as being part of the disease but in most cases does not produce serious problems.

Onset of the disease varies a great deal from childhood to adulthood although almost all individuals will show some signs of the disease by the age of 20 and certainly by 30.

More than any other type of dystrophy, the expression of this disease varies considerably from one person to another, sometimes within the same family. Some may have only mild facial weakness and no more than minimal shoulder weakness all their lives, which may even go unrecognized. About half never have any pelvic girdle weakness that causes them serious problems. However, some, fortunately few, eventually become confined to a wheelchair. Life expectancy in general is not significantly reduced and many remain active throughout their lives. The heart is not affected and there is no intellectual impairment.

This type of dystrophy affects both sexes equally and is inherited as an autosomal dominant trait. The gene has now been located on chromosome 4 and so with appropriate DNA markers it is possible to determine within a family who is likely to carry the affected gene, even though they may be clinically unaffected at the time of examination. From DNA studies it is also possible to get some idea of the likely prognosis in the individual case.

Distal muscular dystrophy

In this type of dystrophy muscle weakness predominantly affects the *distal* limb muscles—those of the forearms and lower legs. But, as in limb girdle muscular dystrophy, there are several other disorders that can also produce this particular distribution of muscle weakness. These include diseases of the spine and spinal cord as well as of the nerves supplying this group of muscles. These possibilities must therefore be excluded before the diagnosis of distal muscular dystrophy can be made.

Weakness in the forearms and hands is present from the beginning and is first noticeable as clumsiness in fine movements, such as fastening buttons, sewing, or typing. Involvement of the lower leg muscles leads to tripping over carpets and steps and makes standing on the heels, or less often on the toes, difficult if not impossible. The proximal limb muscles only occasionally become affected, the disease is slowly progressive, and life span is normal.

This disease, beginning in the twenties or thirties, or even later, appears to be prevalent in Sweden, though cases have now been reported from various other countries throughout the world. It affects both males and females and is inherited as an autosomal dominant trait. However, there are rare types of distal muscular dystrophy that are inherited as autosomal recessive traits. The genes responsible for these various autosomal dominant and autosomal recessive types are now known and therefore DNA studies can help in the diagnosis.

Oculopharyngeal muscular dystrophy

Much of our knowledge of this autosomal dominant disorder has come from studies of French Canadian families with the disease who can be traced back to immigrants from France in 1634. However, the disease is now known to occur also in the USA as well as in Europe.

Onset occurs in the thirties or often later.

As the name implies, the eye muscles are affected early on. At first, movements of the two eyes may be incoordinate and double vision (*diplopia*) can result but is uncommon. Later, weakness of the upper facial muscles develops with drooping of the eyelids, called *ptosis*, which is the most prominent feature of this disease. Mild weakness of the neck muscles and the proximal upper limb muscles commonly occurs. A serious symptom that may develop is difficulty in swallowing, known as *dysphagia*, for which surgery (cricopharyngeal myotomy) may be helpful.

A somewhat similar disease but with earlier onset has been reported in Israel among the Ashkenazim where it is inherited as an autosomal recessive trait.

Recent research has shown that some cases with a similar presentation are proving to have mutations of *mitochondrial* genes. That is, there are mutations of the DNA in the parts of the cell that are important for producing the body's energy. Such subtle differences might seem unimportant—but establishing a precise diagnosis is essential for counselling and the advice of a specialist is particularly important in this form of dystrophy.

Congenital muscular dystrophies

The word congenital simply means 'present at birth'. The congenital muscular dystrophies are therefore a group of dystrophies in which weakness and other problems are evident in the newborn period, or certainly within the first month or so of life. They are inherited as autosomal recessive traits and therefore only affect siblings; parents are perfectly healthy (see Chapter 8).

This is quite a different group of diseases from the so-called *congenital myopathies*. The features of muscle histology seen in congenital myopathies are quite different from those features, characteristic of dystrophy, seen in the congenital muscular dystrophies (Chapter 3). Thus, in any infant who at birth or shortly thereafter appears to be weak (usually expressed at this time as 'floppiness' and feebleness of voluntary movement) a muscle biopsy is important in order to arrive at the correct diagnosis.

About half of all cases of congenital dystrophy have recently been found to be due to a deficiency of a sarcolemmal-associated protein named laminin α_2 or merosin (see Fig. 2.3). This type of dystrophy is relatively severe. Affected children are very floppy (*hypotonic*) at birth and later show generalized muscle wasting and weakness. Joint contractures are also present and these children rarely learn to walk. Furthermore, there is often difficulty in breathing. In fact some form of assisted respiration may be needed, especially in the early stages, and respiratory problems are a frequent cause of mortality. A significant reduction in intelligence is not uncommon in certain forms of this disease. A specific diagnosis of this form of dystrophy, important for genetic counselling and prenatal diagnosis, is based on DNA studies and the histochemistry of muscle tissue.

Remaining cases of congenital dystrophy (often referred to as 'merosin-positive' cases) are very heterogeneous and include several different rare diseases, all of which are also inherited as autosomal recessive traits. However, in general they tend to be less severe and, for example, affected children usually learn to walk, though some rare cases can be associated with learning difficulties and visual problems. Apart from the Fukuyama type of congenital dystrophy, which merits separate consideration, our knowledge of this group of diseases is at present very limited. They are currently the subject of a great deal of research directed at determining their causes.

Fukuyama congenital muscular dystrophy

After Duchenne muscular dystrophy this type of congenital muscular dystrophy is the second most common type of dystrophy in Japan, but seems to be rare outside that country. It is named after Yukio Fukuyama in Tokyo who first described the disease in 1960. The onset is in infancy with generalized muscle weakness and, though able to crawl, few affected children are ever able to walk. Calf pseudohypertrophy is common, and all patients are severely mentally retarded; many also have epilepsy. As in Duchenne muscular dystrophy the serum level of creatine kinase is grossly elevated at first and then gradually declines over the years. Often affected children die in childhood but some survive into their twenties. This type of congenital muscular dystrophy is inherited as an autosomal recessive trait with a 1 in 4 chance of recurrence in subsequent children.

Myotonic dystrophy

This is a unique condition in many ways. First, unlike any other type of dystrophy, *myotonia* is a significant feature—this is the *delayed relaxation* of muscle that occurs after voluntary contraction. Affected people usually refer to this as 'stiffness'. This particularly affects the small muscles of the hands so that after making a fist or gripping an object the muscles relax only slowly. It may be some time before the hand is completely relaxed again, especially in the cold. This is often considered more as a nuisance than as a handicap. This prolonged relaxation can be demonstrated by the doctor by tapping the muscle, whereby the tapped or percussed muscles are seen to contract and then relax only slowly. It can be demonstrated conclusively by electromyography, which is therefore a very important diagnostic test for this disorder.

Secondly, unlike other dystrophies, other organs and tissues are frequently affected. Individuals may develop cataracts as well as various glandular (endocrine) problems—including perhaps a reduction in fertility, increased likelihood of fetal loss (through spontaneous abortions, stillbirths, and deaths in the newborn), and in males early frontal baldness is common. Lethargy and general apathy are also quite common. Children can be severely affected from birth (so-called congenital form) with marked facial weakness, feeding and breathing problems early on, and mental retardation.

Thirdly, the features of muscle histology so characteristic of dystrophy are absent in this condition. Instead, the most prominent characteristic is increased nuclei in the *centre* of muscle fibres, whereas normally they are situated at the periphery of the fibres. Fibre necrosis, phagocytosis, and replacement by fatty connective tissue do not occur.

Despite these differences there are certain similarities with muscular dystrophy, most notably muscle wasting and weakness. This affects the face and neck muscles, lower leg and forearm muscles, and the small muscles of the hands. The heart can also be affected with the development of some degree of heart block. However, unlike the 'true' dystrophies where muscle weakness is the main complaint, myotonic dystrophy is a more generalized disorder.

Only occasionally do all these features of the disease occur in a single person. Sometimes there may be symptomless minute cataracts that are only detected (using a slit lamp) by chance when examining relatives in an affected family. At the other extreme is the congenitally affected infant of an affected mother who often may herself be minimally affected. Children of affected fathers do not have this serious form of the disease.

This disease frequently increases in severity from one generation to the next, a phenomenon referred to as *anticipation*. Thus a grandfather with cataracts and mild myotonia may have a daughter with myotonia and muscle weakness who, in her turn, has a child with the serious congenital form of the disease. This is not uncommon and has now been explained by DNA studies. Such studies can also provide an idea of the possible course of the disease in the individual case.

Though many affected persons have little disability they frequently fail in employment. While the outlook is poor in congenital myotonic dystrophy, adults who are mildly affected with little or no muscle involvement may be expected to survive into middle age and even beyond. The prognosis is worse when there is significant cardiac involvement.

Finally, as in all suspected cases of dystrophy, a careful clinical examination by an experienced physician is essential in establishing the diagnosis. In less severe and minimally affected persons the following tests may be carried out in order to confirm the diagnosis: electromyography to confirm the presence of myotonia, a slit-lamp examination of the eye for the characteristic symptomless multicoloured lens opacities (cataracts) that are often seen early in the disorder, and most importantly DNA studies for the molecular abnormality specific for this disorder.

Other forms of dystrophy

Though the discussion here has centred on the principal clearly defined types of muscular dystrophy, there is little doubt that other types also exist. Some have been given special names, such as the so-called Mabry and Bergia types; others are defined by their apparent distinctive muscle involvement (scapuloperoneal, scapulohumeral) or by their muscle histology (X-linked myopathy and autophagy). But these are rare and in some cases their inclusion as dystrophies is a matter of some dispute among medical scientists. For these reasons they are not discussed here, but details will be found in the major reference texts listed at the end of the book.

5

Treatment

➡ Key points

- Above all, patients and their families should have a positive attitude to the disease. This involves three Ps:

  - promotion and maintenance of good health in general

  - prevention of deformities

  - preservation of respiratory function.

- This means having a good well-balanced diet, avoiding obesity, taking physiotherapy, using special orthoses, and even surgery to correct scoliosis. There are also methods of assisted ventilation that are now available that can transform an individual's life in the later stages of the disease.

- Trials of various drugs in the treatment of dystrophy are nowadays being more carefully designed in order to avoid false claims being made. Prednisone and related steroids may slow down the disease process, at least in the short term, and this is currently being investigated.

- Novel approaches to therapy are now also being considered where the hope is to replace the defective gene by a normal gene. In the long term some form of gene therapy may actually prove to be the best approach, by replacing a diseased gene by its normal equivalent.

- All these developments augur well for patients with muscular dystrophy.

A *cure* for muscular dystrophy would mean replacing the defective causative mutated gene by a normal gene. Since in dystrophy the defective gene is active in every muscle cell of the body as well as in the brain, and in the case of myotonic dystrophy in various other tissues and organs as well, it seemed a forlorn hope that a cure in this sense would ever be possible. The problem seemed insuperable—even to scientists working in the field. Yet very recently there have been technological developments that raise hopes that this might in fact become a distinct possibility, perhaps before not too long. The topic of *gene therapy*, as this is referred to, will be discussed briefly at the end of this chapter.

So, even though there is as yet no cure, a great deal can be done to relieve many of the problems associated with dystrophy and to improve the quality of life. Because of the unrelenting course of muscular dystrophy there was a tendency on the part of healthcare professionals in the past to adopt a somewhat indifferent attitude to treatment. This view is no longer justified. A great deal can be achieved by adopting a positive approach. This positive approach involves three Ps:

♦ promotion and maintenance of good health in general

♦ prevention of deformities through exercises, physiotherapy, orthoses, and surgery

♦ preservation of respiratory function.

Promotion and maintenance of good health

Whatever the type of dystrophy and whatever stage the disease has reached, there are certain general principles always to be considered. Foremost, there is the need to maintain good health in general. A good well-balanced diet with adequate fibre is essential to overcome the common problem of constipation, especially when individuals become immobilized. It is particularly important to prevent weight gain, which often requires professional advice; most muscular dystrophy groups and associations, as well as doctors involved in the disease, can provide helpful information sheets or dietary advice. Plenty of fresh fruit and vegetables are key elements of a good diet. There is no evidence that 'megavitamin' therapy or dietary supplements are of any real value.

Prolonged periods of bed rest after, say, an infection should be discouraged because this may lead to an acceleration of muscle weakness. As a general principle, in the early stages of any of the dystrophies and before walking becomes difficult, individuals should be encouraged to try to lead as normal a life as possible.

Active exercise

A question frequently asked is 'Will exercise improve my muscle strength or slow down the progress of the disease?' The answer is that vigorous or violent exercise or strenuous callisthenics are certainly *not* recommended. They may do actual damage to the muscle and rather than preserving muscle strength, may well have the opposite effect. Severe exercise may also aggravate any heart problems that may be present.

There is no doubt, however, that moderate active forms of exercise do no harm and often have a beneficial psychological effect. Activities of a recreational nature are often preferred and are more likely to be maintained. In this regard swimming is particularly valuable as the buoyancy of the water makes exercises easier to perform, but again it should not be pursued to the point where it becomes exhausting. It is always advisable to have an able-bodied person present at the time just in case any untoward difficulties arise. The best advice is to encourage normal everyday activities wherever possible, supplemented with moderate exercise when this is appropriate and enjoyable.

Passive exercise and physiotherapy

Passive exercise refers to the movement of limbs by another person rather than by the affected individual. The aim is to keep the joints freely mobile and, by *gentle* stretching exercises, to prevent the development of muscle contractures. Parents, partners, and friends can soon learn many of these techniques though it is advisable to have a professional physiotherapist explain and demonstrate the various procedures at the beginning.

> The emphasis is on firmness yet gentleness. *Force must never be used.*

Different techniques are indicated for different problems. Thus in those dystrophies where the heel cords (Achilles tendons) become tight and associated with toe-walking, passive stretching by pushing the foot upwards may be helpful (Fig. 5.1). Passive stretching of the knee and hip joints becomes important after mobility has been lost and where prolonged sitting is leading to contractures of these joints. All such exercises are best carried out on a regular basis at specific times of the day so that they become a routine. After a warm evening bath is a good time for small children. Lyn Hemmings' excellent booklet on

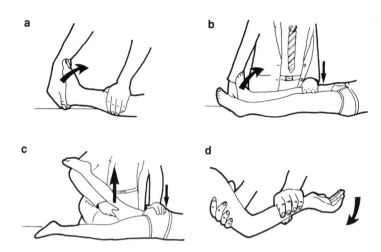

Figure 5.1 Some passive stretching exercises designed to prevent contractures of (a) heel cords (Achilles tendons), (b) knee, (c) hip and (d) elbow joints. (Reproduced with kind permission of Sylvia Hyde.)

the subject is available in the United Kingdom from the Muscular Dystrophy Campaign (see end of book for address).

However, although such exercises may delay the development of contractures, once these occur passive stretching is often ineffective and the use of force can cause serious damage to the muscles and joints. In these circumstances the only solution may be surgery, as will be discussed later.

Some propose the use of night splints in order to help prevent the development of contractures of the ankle and knee joints, but it is very doubtful if such measures have any real value while the individual is still ambulant. They should be measured and fitted by a specialist and must be comfortable to wear, otherwise they are likely to be discarded after a time.

Chronic low-frequency electrical stimulation

There was a great deal of interest a year or two ago in the possible benefits of stimulating weak muscles to contract using low-frequency electrical pulses.

Evidence, however, has shown that this time-consuming and expensive technique is of very doubtful value and cannot be recommended.

Scoliosis

Scoliosis, or curving of the spine to one side, has been mentioned several times. This is a serious problem because it results in compression of the lung on that side, which affects breathing and predisposes to chest infections. This problem rarely arises when individuals are fully mobile—in most cases it only develops once walking and standing are no longer possible and so long periods are spent sitting. A persistently bad sitting position results in the gradual development of spinal curvature.

There are a number of possible ways to impede the development of scoliosis.

◆ It is important to adopt a correct upright sitting position at all times (Fig. 5.2). This sounds much easier than it is, and most of us tend to twist from side to side when sitting. For people with serious muscle weakness this is not easy, or even impossible, and so they tend to adopt a comfortable position and then stay sitting that way.

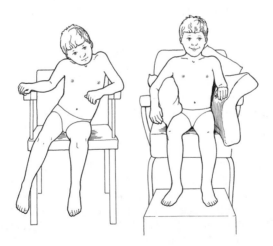

Figure 5.2 (a) A bad sitting position results in the gradual development of spinal curvature. (b) This can be prevented to some extent by sitting upright with the ankles and knees at 90°, on a seat that is firm and not too wide, with the back of the chair upright and the correct position maintained with some form of firm but comfortable support.

- Individually designed firm back supports, body jackets, and braces made of lightweight materials are now available commercially. But although such measures may slow the development of scoliosis, they cannot prevent it, especially in the more rapidly progressive forms of dystrophy, such as Duchenne muscular dystrophy. They are of more benefit to those with relatively benign forms of dystrophy, but whatever the condition, if the spinal curvature progresses beyond about 40° from the vertical, such measures are then impractical and of limited value.

- Other approaches to the problem are to prolong walking by various measures (see below) or resort to surgery.

Prolonging walking

Prolonging walking beyond the point where this is normally no longer possible is a difficult problem, particularly in the more serious forms of dystrophy. It can be achieved by using lightweight plastic or polypropylene splints or *orthoses* that extend from the buttocks down to the ankles, so-called full-length weight-bearing orthoses (Fig. 5.3). If contractures of the heel cords, hips, or knees have already developed, then these must first be dealt with. This often requires an operation and orthoses are then fitted immediately afterwards. Such orthoses can be worn with everyday shoes and underneath trousers.

In Duchenne muscular dystrophy these measures can prolong walking by about 2 years and occasionally for longer, but success depends very much upon the individual. It is not appropriate if the boy is obese or if there is any marked degree of mental handicap, and of course there must be full cooperation. The regime must be started as soon as walking unaided is becoming a serious problem. Once confined to a wheelchair for any period, rehabilitation becomes difficult because of loss of muscle power and also because marked contractures may have developed.

The advantages of this approach include continued independence, easier management by the parents, and, of course, slowing down of the development of contractures and scoliosis. However, some boys and their families find these measures very difficult to cope with. Furthermore, getting about in this way is fraught with problems, not least of which is the need for level surfaces and the tolerance and help of school friends and teachers.

In adults the situation is very different. Here the fitting of various orthoses, coupled with surgery, often proves extremely valuable and may make it possible to continue with gainful employment in an office or similar environment for several years afterwards.

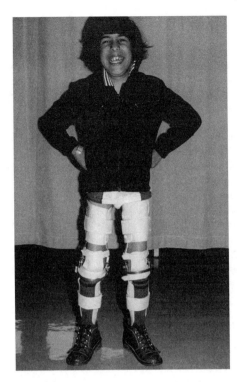

Figure 5.3 Orthoses have to be comfortable.

In the last few years there has been much discussion of the value of *standing frames*. The device is strapped to the body, so enabling the individual to maintain an upright standing position, which otherwise would be impossible. This is only possible, however, if the knee and hips are kept straight by some form of splintage. Wheelchairs can be modified for the same purpose. Such measures are more likely to find use in adults with more slowly progressive forms of dystrophy where they can be of psychological benefit. Maintaining an upright position may also have a beneficial effect on lung function. Some find they can work in this way, for example with a computer or drawing board, for quite long periods of the day.

Aids for the disabled

Many different types of aids for the disabled are now commercially available. Some have been designed for other conditions, such as severe arthritis, but can often be easily modified for people with dystrophy. For example, kitchen aids designed for those with rheumatoid arthritis often prove helpful to those with weakness of their hands due to dystrophy.

Aids range from major modifications to the home (including lifts, ramps, and bathroom fitments) to those which help with mobility (wheelchairs), seating, methods of communication (adapted computers and word processors), and even leisure pursuits (such as gardening). Relevant literature and information is available from the various muscular dystrophy associations and groups listed at the end of the book. A particularly valuable publication is *How to get equipment for disability* by Michael Mandelstam for the Disabled Living Foundation:

Disabled Living Foundation

380–384 Harrow Road

London W9 2 HU

UK

(Tel.: 020 72896111; http://www.dlf.org.uk)

For those who become severely disabled, wheelchair-mounted robotic manipulators and computers are now available. Control panels can be modified to suit individual needs and may permit many everyday activities that otherwise would be impossible. Just what can be accomplished under such circumstances is well illustrated in the case of the world-renowned Professor of Mathematics Stephen Hawking, famous as the author of *A brief history of time*. Such equipment is of course expensive but no doubt with the modification of commercially available equipment this will become less of a problem in future.

> Anything that makes an individual's life more independent and enables the continued pursuit of employment, or even interesting pastimes and hobbies, has to be encouraged.

Perhaps the worst situation of all for those with dystrophy is to feel helpless, worthless, and isolated.

Surgery

At one time there was a vogue for dividing the heel cords in young boys with Duchenne muscular dystrophy, but this and other *early* surgical procedures are now no longer recommended. Not only does it fail to improve muscle strength or walking ability, but the period of bed rest following such surgery may actually be detrimental. Often affected boys are no longer able to walk again following prolonged bed rest.

However, as we have seen, surgical correction of contractures can be valuable in the *later* stages of the disease when walking unaided is becoming increasingly difficult and when it is then designed to prolong ambulation.

Surgery in order to correct scoliosis is also becoming widely accepted. The technique used is referred to as the Luque operation, after Eduardo Luque of Mexico who pioneered the operation. During the operation the spine is straightened as far as possible and the individual vertebrae wired to two stainless steel rods that are thereby fixed to the spine. This produces a rigid and stabilized spine and further curvature is prevented. Postoperative recovery is usually uneventful and requires no more than a week or two in hospital.

Some have advocated this operation as a preventive measure *before* the development of scoliosis, but most agree it is best considered when ambulation has been lost and it is becoming obvious that scoliosis is beginning to develop. The surgeon has to decide, however, if the individual is fit enough for surgery and in particular that lung function is relatively good. The idea is to plan well ahead. If referral is delayed the patient may in fact be found to be unsuitable for surgery.

In Duchenne muscular dystrophy (for which this operation has so far been most used) there is evidence that it helps to preserve lung function and *may* actually prolong life for a few extra years. Certainly, sitting becomes much easier and more comfortable, and in adults with dystrophy there is no doubt that many years of useful and productive life may be made possible in this way.

The decision to undergo surgery requires careful thought and discussion with a surgeon experienced in the disease. No doubt there are advantages but this is a major operation and, like all such operations, carries certain risks that have to be considered.

◆ Increased muscle breakdown results in increased amounts of muscle protein (myoglobin) in the urine, which can sometimes lead to kidney damage.

49

♦ The functioning of the heart may be adversely affected.

♦ There is also the risk of chest infection due to retention of bronchial secretions, resulting from weakness of the respiratory muscles and associated weak cough. Postoperative respiratory care and appropriate physiotherapy are therefore essential.

However, despite these risks—which nowadays are all well recognized by anaesthetists and surgeons—the majority of patients tolerate surgery very well indeed and postoperative recovery is usually uneventful. In several recent large surveys of patients with Duchenne muscular dystrophy who have had major surgery to correct spinal deformities there were very few serious problems. Furthermore, if surgery becomes *necessary* for any reason (for example, cholecystectomy for gall bladder disease), dystrophy in itself should not generally be a reason against having the operation.

In all cases it is essential that the anaesthetist is fully informed of the diagnosis *before* any procedures are undertaken. As we say, 'forewarned is to be forearmed', and in this way any problems that might arise during surgery will either be prevented from happening or recognized as soon as they occur and then treated immediately before complications develop.

As not all hospital nursing staff will have come across a patient with muscular dystrophy before, in order to help them know what a particular patient can do, it is useful to have a 'hospital card' that records the diagnosis and what the patient can do physically in regard to feeding and toilet arrangements. The Muscular Dystrophy Campaign of Great Britain, for example, makes such cards available for patients who may be planning to go into hospital.

Fractures

Because of their muscle weakness, some people with dystrophy frequently sustain bone fractures as a result of minor accidents such as falling. This is partly due to the fact that the long bones of the limbs are often less strong than normal due to disuse. Because of the adverse effects of prolonged immobilization on muscle function, fractures are often treated with minimal splintage so that mobility can be resumed as soon as possible. Otherwise fractures in patients with dystrophy present no additional problems: they heal normally and call for no special orthopaedic measures.

Respiratory problems

Not only does chest deformity restrict airflow on the compressed side, but respiratory problems are also aggravated by weakness of the respiratory muscles themselves. Simple non-invasive tests of lung function that can be carried out every 6 months if necessary are now available, and in this way any significant impairment can be detected early before serious problems might arise. In Duchenne muscular dystrophy, for example, from about age 10 there is a gradual deterioration in lung function. In the less severe forms of dystrophy the effects on respiratory function are less marked but they nevertheless occur. In fact, impaired pulmonary function and respiratory failure are major causes of illness and death in most types of dystrophy. Preservation of lung function and the prevention and treatment of chest infections are therefore among the most important aspects of the treatment of patients with dystrophy.

Do not smoke

At the simplest level parents, partners, relatives, and friends should be dissuaded from smoking in the same room as an affected individual. Apart from perhaps those with the distal and oculopharyngeal types of dystrophy where lung function is not affected, people with dystrophy *should never smoke*, particularly cigarettes. I am all too aware that such advice is sometimes hard to accept. Nevertheless, it cannot be emphasized too strongly that not smoking is one of the most important things that people with dystrophy can do for themselves to help preserve their lung function.

Respiratory tract infections

Many advocate vaccination against influenza at the beginning of the winter months and *all* infections of the respiratory tract must be treated *thoroughly*, with a course of antibiotics where necessary. Even seemingly mild chest infections should never be ignored. In those who are at all severely affected and where there is already some breathing difficulty, hospitalization should be considered for any respiratory infection.

Postural drainage

Any attempt to impede the development of scoliosis will have a beneficial effect on respiratory function. Deep breathing exercises can help (Fig. 5.4). Parents, partners, and friends can also be instructed in how to carry out the procedure of so-called *postural drainage*, which helps to remove the accumulation of mucus secretions in the lungs, which, because of a weak cough, can be a

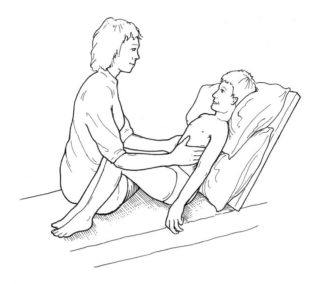

Figure 5.4 Deep breathing: the helper's hands apply gentle pressure over the lower part of the rib cage while the person breathes in as much as possible, trying to move the ribs outwards against the hands, and the breath is then held for a few seconds before breathing out. This should be repeated, say, 10 times at each session.

problem in those who are more severely affected (this is not usually necessary in those who are fully ambulant). In postural drainage the head has to be lower than the chest to encourage drainage and this can be achieved by lying face down with a pillow under the hips or by lying flat, face down, and raising the foot of the bed (Fig. 5.5). With a slightly cupped hand, the lower part of the chest is clapped and the patient encouraged to cough at the same time, if this is possible. The mucus secretions that drain into the throat can then be removed, with suction apparatus if necessary. To be effective this technique is best if first learned from a doctor or physiotherapist who can demonstrate exactly how the clapping should be carried out and which positions are best adopted by a particular patient in order to encourage the drainage of secretions that may have accumulated.

Assisted ventilation

Despite rigorous treatment of all chest infections and of scoliosis by surgery if necessary, in more severe cases lung function will inevitably decline as the

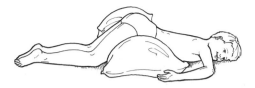

Figure 5.5 Postural drainage: the person is placed face down with the head lower than the chest.

muscles of respiration become increasingly affected. Lung function tests will of course detect these changes. However, there are certain symptoms that are a warning of an impending serious decline in lung function. Normally when we sleep our breathing becomes slower and shallower. In dystrophy respiration may be quite adequate during the day but become so inadequate at night that there is very poor oxygenation of the blood and so-called *nocturnal hypoxia* develops. Symptoms that indicate that this is developing and that respiratory function is therefore becoming seriously affected include:

◆ restless sleep

◆ nightmares

◆ morning confusion

◆ headache

◆ drowsiness during the day.

Later, more obvious signs of poor lung function become evident with increasing breathlessness and difficulty speaking. If symptoms suggestive of nocturnal hypoxia develop, medical attention should be sought and, if confirmed, *assisted ventilation* may be necessary. A number of methods are available, referred to as negative and positive pressure ventilators. The former includes the *cuirass* or body shell, such as the Tunnicliffe jacket for example. These jackets consist of a rigid shell that encloses but does not touch the chest wall and abdomen. The shell is covered by an airtight jacket to which negative pressure is applied. Other jackets employ alternating positive pressure, but all have the disadvantages of being difficult to put on and cold to wear at night.

Positive pressure ventilators provide ventilation through non-invasive positive pressure ventiliation (NPPV) or bi-level positive airway pressure (BiPaP). Of all methods the most favoured is to use an *intermittent positive pressure ventilator* connected to a nasal tube, mouth adaptor, or facial mask, depending on individual preference. This is the most efficient way of artificial ventilation as it provides a fixed volume of inspired air and then allows passive expiration. At first this may only be necessary during or immediately after an acute respiratory infection or later on at night, when it can transform an individual's life. On questioning, most of those on this form of intermittent ventilation say that it has definitely improved the quality of their lives. Unfortunately, lung function often continues to deteriorate, necessitating ever longer periods of ventilation.

Eventually, which may be several years later in some cases, *a tracheostomy* may have to be considered. This involves inserting a tube into the windpipe (trachea) just below the 'Adam's apple'. This is usually done under local anaesthesia. The tube is then connected to a ventilator.

Tracheostomy sometimes has to be performed as an emergency procedure during an acute and severe respiratory infection in order to ensure adequate respiration and so that secretions can be removed by suction directly from the upper airways. However, having once started this means of ventilation it may later prove difficult to wean the patient off the machine.

In recent times there has been increasing interest in *elective* tracheostomy, that is, carrying out the procedure as a means of ensuring adequate lung function for the future and not as a response to acute infection, but this raises serious problems of maintenance and nursing care that need to be carefully considered. Nevertheless, an increasing number of patients are now being managed in this way. With a tracheostomy and assisted ventilation, boys with Duchenne dystrophy, for example, now survive into their third decade.

Heart problems

In those disorders in which heart block is a particular problem, such as Emery–Dreifuss dystrophy and myotonic dystrophy, regular ECG (EKG) or echocardiographic examination is important in order to detect the problem early on. Specific treatment may then be indicated and a permanent pacemaker may have to be considered. The decision whether or not to insert a pacemaker rests very much on the cardiologist in discussion with the patient.

Long-term preventive treatment, with digitalis compounds for example, has no value. However, in the later stages of dystrophy when heart involvement may become evident, conventional treatment with appropriate drugs is indicated as would be the case in anyone with heart disease.

Drug treatment

In myotonic dystrophy there are certain drugs that can be used to treat myotonia on the rare occasions when this is troublesome. These include *quinine* and *procainamide*, but because the former often produces a disturbing ringing in the ears (tinnitus) and both may adversely affect the heart in myotonic dystrophy, the drug *diphenylhydantoin* is now preferred. Caution should be exercised in taking the drug during pregnancy, however, because of the risk of inducing cleft lip and palate in the fetus. Though this is relatively small, even a small risk is important when the symptom being treated is relatively benign and may not have really warranted treatment in the first place.

For other types of dystrophy, no drug has yet been found that significantly improves muscle strength in the long term. In the past many have been tried and claimed to be beneficial (Table 5.1), but with subsequent carefully controlled trials this optimism has invariably proved to be ill-founded. There are a number of reasons for this. The diagnosis may not have been precise and the inclusion, for example, of cases of Becker muscular dystrophy in a study of the effects of a drug on Duchenne muscular dystrophy could have given the mistaken impression of slowing the course of the disease. As various dystrophies often show periods of *apparent* arrest or slowing of the disease process, this too could be misinterpreted as being due to the drug being used. Overenthusiasm by the investigator, coupled with understandable optimism on the part of those treated, may also influence the interpretation of the results of a drug trial. For these and for various other reasons a trial of any therapy must be very carefully designed and executed.

1. A *precise diagnosis* must be established in all those included in the trial.
2. *Objective* means of determining any improvement must be used. For example, muscle strength may be assessed using a special measuring instrument called a *myometer*.
3. An *adequate number* of people must be included in the trial in order that any results may be statistically valid.

4. Most importantly, in order to avoid any bias in the interpretation of results, all studies should be *carefully controlled*. That is, the patients should be divided into two groups that are matched exactly for age, sex, and severity of the disease. One group is then given the active drug (the treated group) and the other group (the control group) is given a *placebo* (an inactive compound that closely resembles the active drug, both in appearance and texture). This approach is not restricted to drugs to be taken by mouth, however, but could equally apply to other trials. For example, with injected drugs the control group might be injected with normal saline solution.

5. Such trials should be *double-blind*. This means that neither the patient and family nor the investigator know who is taking the active drug and who is taking the placebo; the code is maintained by an uninvolved third party, usually the pharmacist. After a suitable period, at least 6 months and often longer, the code is broken and the two groups are carefully compared for any differences.

Table 5.1 Some drugs that have been used in various therapeutic trials, mainly in Duchenne muscular dystrophy: none have proven in clinical trials to be significantly effective

Drug	Basis for use	First reported trial
Allopurinol	Increases nucleotide formation, believed to be depleted in dystrophic muscle	1976
Amino acids	Deficiency of muscle proteins	1953
Aminoglycoside antibiotics	Suppress gene mutation	1999
Anabolic steroids	Anabolic effect	1955
Aspirin, propranolol, etc.	Counteract proposed defect in biogenic amine metabolism	1977
Azathioprine	Immunosuppression	1993
Calcium blockers	Reduce muscle intracellular calcium	1982
Catecholamines	Counteract proposed defect in muscle sympathetic innervation	1930
Coenyzme Q	Possible benefit in murine dystrophy	1974
Creatine	Deficiency in muscle	2000

(continued)

Table 5.1 Some drugs that have been used in various therapeutic trials, mainly in Duchenne muscular dystrophy: none have proven in clinical trials to be significantly effective (*continued*)

Drug	Basis for use	First reported trial
Dantrolene	Inhibits release of calcium from sarcoplasmic reticulum	1983
Digitalis and other cardiac glycosides	Prevent progressive cardiomyopathy	1963
Glycine	Believed to stimulate muscle creatine synthesis	1932
Growth hormone	Anabolic effects	1973
Growth hormone inhibitor	Growth hormone deficiency ameliorates disease	1984
Ketoacids	Reduce muscle protein degradation	1982
Leucine	Increases protein synthesis	1984
Nucleotides (e.g. laevadosin)	Replacement of nucleotides believed to be depleted in dystrophic muscle	1960
Oestrogens	Anabolic effect	1972
Oxandrolone	Anabolic effect	1997
Pancreatic extract	Possible benefit in murine dystrophy	1976
Penicillamine	Possible benefit in avian dystrophy	1977
Prednisone	Anabolic effect	1974
Protease inhibitors	Possible benefit in murine dystrophy	1984
Superoxide dismutase	Removal of superoxide radicals associated with membrane damage	1980
Testosterone	Anabolic effect	1955
Thyroxine	Thyroxine depresses creatine phosphokinase	1964
Vasodilators	Counteract proposed defect in muscle microcirculation	1963
Vitamin B_6	Vitamin B_6-deficient rats develop a myopathy	1940
Vitamin E	Vitamin E-deficient animals develop a myopathy	1940
Zinc	Membrane 'stabilizer'	1986

This has only been a somewhat superficial review of the design of treatment trials and further details can be found in many modern texts. In 1984 a colloquium was held in Bangor, Pennsylvania, USA sponsored by the Muscular Dystrophy Association of America, which addressed many of the problems involved in drug trials, particularly in Duchenne muscular dystrophy. The Proceedings have been published and provide much useful information and guidance (*Muscle and Nerve* 1985; **8**: 451–92).

If you are wondering why this topic has been discussed in such detail, the reason is that all too often in the past ill-designed studies have led to spurious claims being made for the effectiveness of particular treatments. This still occurs today, though the majority of responsible investigators are now well aware of the need for carefully designed studies in order to prevent this happening. Raising false hopes in those with a disease such as muscular dystrophy is inexcusable.

Current approaches to treatment are the use of the drug prednisone and related compounds and gene therapy.

Prednisone

In the last few years therapeutic trials have concentrated on two major groups of drugs: 'calcium blockers' and prednisone and its related compounds. The reason behind testing the former was that the inflow of calcium into muscle fibres has been shown to be an important factor in muscle damage in dystrophy (see Chapter 2). Unfortunately, not only have carefully controlled trials failed to show any beneficial effects of these drugs, but we now know that they can have severe side-effects in dystrophy. The story regarding prednisone is more promising and encouraging.

The value of prednisone in the treatment of dystrophy was first considered over 30 years ago. Recent studies show that it does lead to improvement in muscle strength, at least in the short term and can prolong walking by 2-4 years. The long-term effects are more problematical, and this drug can have undesirable side-effects (including mood changes, weight gain and suppression of the immune system). One possibility, currently advocated, is to use a steroid on alternate days as means of reducing possible side-effects. Compounds related to prednisone but with fewer side-effects are also being studied. Parents of boys with Duchenne dystrophy considering the possibility of treatment with steroids should first discuss this with their family doctor and hospital specialist, as such treatment requires careful supervision and monitoring by those experienced in the field.

Meanwhile, as we understand more of the detail of the biochemical processes that lead to muscle weakness in dystrophy, it may be possible to select or even design a drug that influences or interrupts these processes. In this way progressive weakness may be slowed, arrested, or even reversed. But it is also possible that an effective treatment might still be found by chance. The history of medicine is full of such examples, and there will always be a place for clever and original ideas in finding a drug treatment for dystrophy.

Gene therapy

At the beginning of this chapter we mentioned that until very recently the idea of compensating for a defective mutant gene by adding a normal gene seemed quite unrealistic, and seemed more in the realms of science fiction. But this is no longer so. Though the particulars of the complex technology need not concern us too much, a few details may convey some of its exciting potential.

First, DNA is extracted from, say, white blood cells of a normal healthy individual; the particular gene of interest is then isolated from this DNA. In the case of the very large dystrophin gene, only the most important part (so-called mini-dystrophin gene) is used.

Secondly, for a gene to be active and so synthesize a specific protein in a particular tissue (for example, dystrophin in muscle) it is also necessary to include along with the gene a *promoter*, a sequence of DNA that ensures that the gene is 'turned on' in the appropriate tissue. The promoter and associated gene are then *cloned*, a process whereby a micro-organism is induced to synthesize millions of copies. The cloned gene with its promoter is then transferred to the patient in the hope that it will take over from the defective mutant gene and so synthesize the particular protein that is absent or abnormal in the patient. There are several ways in which genes can be transferred.

In the case of muscular dystrophy the simplest way would be to inject the cloned mini-dystrophin gene *directly* into the patient's muscle. This has been shown to work in dystrophic mice but the results indicate that the technique as used so far is not very efficient. Only a very small proportion of the muscle fibres in injected animals appear to synthesize dystrophin. A method has to be found to increase the efficiency of the system if sufficient fibres are to be induced to synthesize enough dystrophin to be clinically effective. But there is considerable potential in this approach because animal experiments have now shown that DNA can also be injected directly into the heart of the affected animals. Dystrophin synthesis then occurs in this tissue as well.

Yet another way to transfer a gene is to use a virus as a carrier or vector. Here some of the genes of the virus are replaced by a normal human gene and a promoter and then the virus is used as a vehicle to convey them to the patient. Of course the virus has to be 'disarmed' or 'crippled' in some way so that it is no longer infectious, but there are relatively straightforward ways of doing this. In fact the replacement of a large part of the virus's own genes by human DNA ensures that the engineered virus is unable to divide and be infectious. This approach is currently being used to treat, for example, certain genetic diseases that affect the immune system. With regard to muscular dystrophy, experiments have shown that when a virus carrying a mini-dystrophin gene and promoter are injected into affected mice, in some experiments up to 90 per cent of the muscle fibres subsequently synthesize dystrophin.

Some investigators are attempting to block or circumvent the particular mutation in the dystrophin gene. This involves specially synthesized so-called oligonucleotides that bypass it during the process of protein synthesis, referred to as exon skipping.

This approach, using so-called anti-sense oligonucleotides, is currently undergoing preliminary clinical trials and its advocates are hopeful of success. An allied technique is to use a novel drug that bypasses an abnormal 'stop' codon within a gene. This technique augurs well, but in this case would only be applicable to those 10 per cent of boys with Duchenne dystrophy who have such a 'stop' codon as the cause of their problem. Yet another approach to the problem currently attracting a great deal of attention is to increase the synthesis ('upregulation') of a muscle protein that can compensate for the deficiency of, say, dystrophin. This might then be expected to effect a treatment. Recent experiments indicate that upregulation of muscle utrophin (a protein much like dystrophin) leads to amelioration of the disease in the dystrophic mouse. Unfortunately, the upregulation of utrophin in mice was achieved by molecular biological techniques not possible in humans. In human dystrophy there is much interest in finding a drug or other compound that will upregulate utrophin. An entirely different approach is to extract from a healthy donor a sample of muscle cells from which are derived so-called *stem cells*. These are cells that have the capability, when injected into the affected recipient, to grow into normal functioning muscle. The technology is difficult but its advocates are also hopeful of finding this an effective treatment.

So far much research in this field has involved animal studies. The hope is that the technology will prove to be safe as well as effective in treatment. This technology also opens up the possibility of perhaps one day even treating the affected fetus in the womb before birth—but we are still a very long way from this.

Patients and therapeutic trials

With perhaps the exception of some surgical procedures, as we have seen, all therapeutic trials, where practicable, should include controls. In a double-blind study this means that some patients will be allocated to the control group with a placebo or some form of sham treatment. If there is no evidence before the trial to suggest that the proposed therapy has any beneficial effect, the possibility of being placed in the control group will be acceptable. But if there is any suggestion at all that the treatment could be effective there is sometimes an understandable resentment that a participant in the trial might be included in a control group. After all, this would mean being denied treatment for as long as the study lasts. The reassurance that one can give is that the investigator would be the first to offer the treatment to all his or her patients if, on breaking the code, the results showed that it was at all effective. A possible solution to this problem is to compare the course of the disease in patients being treated with the *expected* course, known from past studies of untreated patients—*natural history controls*.

Another sort of problem that can occur in a therapeutic trial was brought home to me personally a few years ago. We were engaged in a double-blind controlled study of a calcium-blocker drug in Duchenne muscular dystrophy. After a year we noticed that several boys were developing some unexpected heart problems. This forced us to break the code, only to discover that these boys were all taking the active drug and not the placebo. Furthermore, on analysing the results the drug was shown not to be significantly affecting the course of the disease. For both these reasons we decided to abandon the trial. But we met with very stiff opposition from some of the parents who were by then firmly convinced that the drug was having a beneficial effect (although they did not know if their son was on the drug) and wanted to continue with the trial. This was a very upsetting time for all of those involved until we were able to convince the parents of the scientific validity of our findings.

For all these reasons, the decision to participate in a therapeutic trial needs to be thought about very carefully beforehand. All the pros and cons should be discussed with the clinical staff involved as well as, if possible, an independent medical adviser who is also experienced in muscular dystrophy. In this way the patient, or the parents in the case of a child, will be better able to make a reasoned decision as to whether or not to participate. If there is any doubt, these doubts should be expressed. Medical staff will respect such feelings and there is nothing to stop an individual changing his or her mind later about taking part in a trial at some future date.

6

Living with muscular dystrophy

➡ Key points

♦ The coping process, following a stressful event, occurs in five stages:
(1) shock and denial; (2) anxiety; (3) anger and guilt; (4) depression;
(5) psychological homeostasis.

♦ The emotional and psychological effects of dystrophy on the affected
person as well as on the family are often suppressed and ignored.
Individuals vary in their response. Some adapt very well but others
may withdraw and become isolated and depressed. The relationship
between the parents of an affected child may suffer. They have to
learn to share responsibilities and often need time for each other so
that their own relationship does not deteriorate. When there is already
a family history of the disorder, relatives may well be able to provide
additional support and comfort.

♦ Affected people themselves often harbour feelings of poor self-esteem
and fears about the progressive nature of the disease and its prognosis.
Sexual problems may also arise.

♦ It should not be assumed that the unaffected brothers and sisters of
an affected child, or the children of an affected parent, are emotionally
unscathed. They often have their own emotional problems in response
to the disease.

♦ There is no simple answer to all these matters, but open and frank
discussions with relatives, friends, and professionals involved in
dystrophy are often helpful. Voicing fears and concerns often helps to
resolve them.

A detailed examination of all the possible social and psychological effects of living with dystrophy is beyond the scope of this little book whose emphasis is more on medical problems and their management. But as the subject is so very important, some indications of the sort of problems that may occur, along with their possible solutions, will be discussed. Much more detailed treatment will be found in some of the specialized texts listed at the end of the book.

When and how much to tell

An intelligent affected child will no doubt sooner or later become aware of his or her problem. With children it is probably not a good idea to discuss the full implications of the diagnosis at the beginning. In many ways it is best to encourage questions and to answer them sensibly and honestly, in a way appropriate to the age and level of understanding. The best way is to provide a little information at a time and as often as questions and opportunities arise.

The natural inclination for most parents is to shield their affected son or daughter from what they themselves perceive as a cruel blow, and they respond by being overprotective. This should be avoided as much as possible otherwise feelings of independence that normally surface around adolescence may be stifled and the resulting frustration lead to more stress within the family.

> It is important that affected persons at any age never feel overprotected.

They should be encouraged, within the limits of their disabilities of course, to feel free to enlarge their social contacts and circle of friends.

In the case of adults, more and detailed information can be provided from the beginning. However, there is always a need to be guided by the person's questions and their response. To go into too much detail about the ultimate outcome could prove very distressing. On the other hand, some people may be quite willing to accept such information in order to plan for the future with regard to housing and employment, for example. As in all other emotionally charged situations, tactful questioning can often indicate how far to proceed, and open and frank discussions are invariably helpful.

Individual responses

As the psychological effects of dystrophy (or for that matter any disabling condition) are often suppressed or concealed, it is easy to believe that they do not exist. Most affected people give every impression of being well adapted and having come to terms with their disability. In some cases this may well be true, but in others it would be entirely wrong to assume that they are emotionally and psychologically unscathed by the disease. Several studies have shown that feelings of isolation, inadequacy, and worthlessness are often harboured. Furthermore, needs for privacy, affection, and sexual satisfaction may never be expressed.

As with any of life's major events, not everyone reacts in the same way. This is certainly true in dystrophy. Even affected brothers may each respond differently to their increasing physical disability. In a family with Becker muscular dystrophy which I know one affected brother in his thirties seems to have come to terms with his problems, is happily married, and gainfully employed in an office environment. His brother, a year or two older, seems never to have accepted his disability and remains isolated and depressed. He has never married and has not worked for several years. The former has effectively adapted to his problems, whereas the latter has withdrawn because to him the situation appears hopeless.

Commonly, those affected often feel physically unattractive and if, at the same time, there is any intellectual impairment they may well feel inferior and as a result become depressed. However, major depressive illness is uncommon. In some the response to the disease is reflected in serious behavioural problems.

Although some deny that their inability to find sexual satisfaction is a cause of distress, to others this can be a problem, particularly in the more slowly progressive forms of dystrophy that begin in adolescence or later. It is also quite a common problem in boys with Duchenne muscular dystrophy as they approach adolescence.

Quite apart from these sorts of emotional responses to physical handicap, which will vary from one individual to another, there are others of a more *social* nature, which in their turn may also produce psychological reactions. Physical disability may be viewed as a social stigma and become a source of embarrassment to the entire family. In fact the psychological and social consequences of dystrophy almost always involve other family members to varying degrees. The impact of the disease is very rarely, if ever, limited to the affected people themselves.

In order to do anything about these problems it is first necessary to recognize and accept that they do exist. Let us begin at the beginning when the diagnosis is first made.

The coping process

Because dystrophy often begins in a vague and ill-defined way there may be some delay before the diagnosis is made, which I am afraid, is still often the case in Duchenne muscular dystrophy. However, this should become less of a problem as family doctors increasingly become aware of the possibility of dystrophy in young boys with a walking problem. But this delay often means that the parents may have been suspicious that something was seriously wrong for some time. When the diagnosis is made and the nature of the disease explained, then inevitably the parents of an affected child, or the patients themselves in late-onset dystrophies, will experience shock and often disbelief.

> 'Why has this happened to us?'; 'It can't be true, he is so well and no one else in the family is affected'; 'I have never had a day's illness in my life until now. How can it be muscular dystrophy?'; and so on.

The psychological sequence of events that occurs following any stressful event, such as when the diagnosis of a serious disease like dystrophy is first made, is referred to as the coping process. It also occurs, for example, after divorce or during bereavement.

This sequence of events has been much described by psychologists and five sequential stages are recognized.

The duration of each stage varies from one person to another. Some may eventually reach the stage of depression only to return for a time to the first stage. Very rarely, a parent, or even an affected person, may never progress beyond the first stage. They never accept that their child is affected or that they themselves are affected.

Shock and denial

At this stage there is often denial that anything untoward is wrong. That is why it is so important that no discussion of diagnostic possibilities should take place until all the necessary investigations have been completed (Chapter 3). The paediatrician or physician can *then* with confidence explain what the diagnosis is and what the outcome is likely to be. Any discussion of the various possibilities before a definitive diagnosis has been established could be confusing and ultimately prove misleading. For these reasons it is therefore unwise to pressurize the paediatrician or physician into giving a diagnosis before all the investigations are complete.

Anxiety

At this stage the situation has been accepted but now anxiety about the future begins to emerge. Judgement and reason are often impaired and therefore firm decisions about the future should be delayed. A major decision taken at this time about family planning or housing, for example, is likely to be too influenced by the trauma of events to be rational. The situation needs to be carefully assessed before any major decisions are made, and this will require long discussions with a counsellor who can provide emotional support. This stage usually precedes, but on occasion may follow, the next stage.

Anger and guilt

This is perhaps the most difficult stage of all. Parents or the patient may feel anger towards the physician or counsellor. Parents may be resentful if, for example, they were never offered prenatal diagnosis so that it could have been prevented. An adult may be angry that the diagnosis was not made sooner. Very often parents and patients blame themselves and harbour serious feelings of guilt. In X-linked recessive disorders, such as Duchenne muscular dystrophy, which are transmitted by females who carry the disease but are themselves unaffected (Chapter 8), mothers may feel especially guilty. Fathers may also harbour such feelings. To the outsider this may all seem quite irrational, but to parents under stress these can be very real problems. Careful understanding and sympathetic counselling are essential.

Depression

At this stage the situation has been completely accepted: the diagnosis is clear, and the course and prognosis are understood. The result is then often a feeling of depression. Rarely is this profound and sufficient to require treatment. Usually it is more a general feeling of low spirits. It is probably only when this stage has been reached that meaningful discussions about the future are possible. Discussions about family planning or prenatal diagnosis, for example, can now be made.

Homeostasis

This term implies normality and at this stage the emotional response to the disease is now believed to have returned to normal. But it is doubtful if this stage is ever really reached. There will inevitably always be a sense of loss and deprivation throughout life.

When there is a family history

In late-onset dystrophies some unaffected family members may harbour deep-seated anxieties throughout childhood and adulthood that they may also become affected. In the case of Becker muscular dystrophy, for example, a creatine phosphokinase test will be helpful in resolving the problem, but in other disorders more investigative tests may be necessary. These may include DNA studies and also, in myotonic dystrophy, electromyography and slit-lamp examination (Chapter 4). The possibility that such fears may exist should never be dismissed lightly. They are often not expressed openly, and direct and careful questioning by a parent or partner may be necessary to elicit the admission that such fears exist. In many such cases complete reassurance is possible.

There is, however, one positive aspect of having a family history of dystrophy. Parents and partners may benefit from the advice and support of relatives who have already had experience of the disease. In some communities where families are closely knit and family ties are strong, this can work to considerable advantage. But unfortunately nowadays families are often dispersed and such close support is not possible. Occasionally relatives may not wish to share their experiences and anxieties with others in the family because of embarrassment or for other reasons. Their views have to be respected.

The affected person

Above all, the affected person, whether a child or adult, should be allowed to talk about his or her frustrations, disappointments, and anxieties for the future. As Ian Pullen, a psychiatrist experienced in the field, has written about Duchenne muscular dystrophy:

> Many people, including parents do not allow the child to talk about these areas for fear of putting ideas into his head. The ideas certainly are there already but most children are denied the opportunity of communicating them to others. This may make them feel more isolated and abnormal because it prevents others from empathizing accurately with their position.

Furthermore, about one-third of parents of boys with Duchenne muscular dystrophy whom Pullen interviewed had great difficulty even talking to each other about the disease.

In the case of people with late-onset types of dystrophy, partners also often complain that there is a lack of communication.

All experts in the field now agree that frank and open discussions with parents or with partners are to be encouraged. If this is not possible, for whatever reason, then such discussions should take place with a professional counsellor or similar person who has had wide experience of the disease.

So far we have been discussing these problems in generalities, but some problems are particularly important in certain types of dystrophy. For example, we have seen (Chapter 5) that there are advantages to be gained from prolonging walking beyond the point when this might normally be lost, and that this can be achieved by surgery and by fitting various orthoses. However, boys with Duchenne muscular dystrophy may not wish to have surgery and their wishes must be respected. Or later they may find that walking with full-length orthoses is too difficult, and they feel insecure and frightened of falling. In these circumstances it would be unkind and perhaps even harmful to persist. Another significant period in the course of Duchenne muscular dystrophy is when surgery may be contemplated in order to prevent scoliosis and impede any deterioration in lung function (Chapter 5). There is only a relatively brief period when this can be done—when walking unaided has become impossible and before significant spinal curvature and deterioration in lung function has occurred. This 'window of opportunity' only lasts perhaps 1 or 2 years and forces the parents and child to confront the disease in a way they have not had to do in the past. Difficult decisions have to be made during this short time and the strain on all concerned can be considerable. Open discussions some time beforehand are often helpful. These discussions could involve another family that has already gone through this difficult decision-making period in the past.

Psychosexual problems

The existence of psychosexual problems in the disabled was often ignored or dismissed by many professionals in the past—but attitudes are changing. After adolescence many boys with Duchenne muscular dystrophy appear not to be distressed by sexual problems, while others become frustrated in their inability to find sexual satisfaction. Physical disability may actually preclude any relief they might obtain from masturbation. In adults with dystrophy these problems often become magnified. Not only may they feel physically unattractive and have a poor body image, but there may be very limited opportunities for mixing with people of the opposite sex. This, however, is now becoming less of a problem with social clubs designed for the physically disabled.

After meeting a partner there may be problems of impotence and infertility, as in myotonic dystrophy. In other types of dystrophy the main problem may be the actual physical act of intercourse because of muscle weakness. Sympathetic discussions with a mature counsellor experienced in such matters often help a great deal. Useful contacts are given at the end of the book.

Effects on the parents

When a child is diagnosed as having muscular dystrophy, usually Duchenne muscular dystrophy, the effects on the parents are, of course, devastating. As we have seen they cope by gradually adapting to the fact that the child has a serious and progressive disease for which at present there is no cure. But they also have to realize that this is likely to affect their own relationships with each other.

Understandably, one parent, usually the mother, will have to devote a great deal of time to caring for her affected son, especially when walking becomes significantly affected. The other parent, usually the father, may be excluded from this caring because he is absent at work during the day. As a result the mother may feel overburdened by the problem which she may feel should be shared more. In addition, she may also feel isolated from her friends and neighbours by having an affected son. The extra attention given to the son may make his father feel rejected and isolated. This often goes unrecognized because many men are reluctant to reveal their feelings.

For whatever reason, parents may find they have little opportunity to be together or to have a holiday. Furthermore, the very real fear of perhaps having another affected son may seriously affect their sexual relationship. In one survey half the couples had serious marital problems and a quarter had separated. What can be done about this?

Parents should realize from the very beginning that these sorts of problems can occur and are quite common. Again, open and frank discussions between themselves, perhaps with other similarly affected families or with a counsellor, can often be helpful. Couples have to accept that caring has to be shared and that neither should feel rejected by the other partner. On a purely practical level, couples should find a mature and reliable babysitter and be encouraged to go out together at least once a week. A mother or partner might consider part-time employment as a change of environment and should not feel guilty in doing so. After all, they are then more likely to feel refreshed and cope better with their responsibilities.

A definitive approach to contraception (such as tubal ligation or vasectomy) often removes fears of pregnancy and makes the sexual relationship once more a relaxed and enjoyable experience. To others sexual abstinence may be the only acceptable solution.

Having said all this it has to be remembered that many couples cope extremely well. An affected child may actually have the effect of bringing parents and the family closer together. I am repeatedly touched by the sensitive and loving relationship I come across between an affected person and his or her caring partner. There is no doubt that to some the experience of having an affected child or partner brings out their best qualities.

Effects on unaffected siblings

In Duchenne muscular dystrophy an unaffected brother may well worry that he too will become affected. This possibility should never be ignored and the solution is to have a creatine phosphokinase test (Chapter 3) with complete reassurance when this is found to be normal. Apart from the often unexpressed fear that they might also become affected like their brother or sister, siblings often feel isolated and ignored. Though parents may try to be even-handed to all their children, inevitably the affected child will warrant more attention. In this way unaffected brothers and sisters may feel neglected or even jealous or resentful. When these feelings are admitted the unaffected sibling may increasingly feel shame and guilt.

Irwin Siegel, an expert in this field, suggests that unaffected siblings should be encouraged to think about their attitudes to their affected brother. He lists a number of questions that they should discuss with their father or mother, teacher, doctor, social worker, or psychologist. Apart from questions about the disease itself, some others are:

1. Are you afraid of ever asking questions about muscular dystrophy? Why?
2. How would life be different for you if you didn't have a disabled brother?
3. Does he worry you? In what ways?
4. Do you ever feel that your brother always gets what he wants because he is ill and you aren't?
5. How is life different in your house than in homes where there is not a child who is disabled?

6. Is more expected of you at home because your brother is disabled?

7. How do you feel your parents should act towards your disabled brother or towards you?

8. Are you ever angry about the fact that your brother has muscular dystrophy? Why?

9. How are you different from your friends who don't have a brother with muscular dystrophy?

10. What concerns you most about your brother's muscular dystrophy?

At least such questions help to concentrate the mind on the possible concerns and anxieties that an unaffected brother or sister may be harbouring. As in all problems of an emotional or psychological nature associated with dystrophy, open discussion can often prove beneficial. Allaying fears and anxieties among their unaffected children, as well as reassuring them of their love and affection, are essential responsibilities of parents with an affected child.

Effects on the children of an affected parent

In many respects the emotional and psychological effects of having a parent seriously affected with dystrophy are not unlike those faced by the unaffected brothers or sisters of a boy with Duchenne muscular dystrophy. There may be fears that they too may become affected, and they may even come to resent the attention being bestowed on their disabled parent to their exclusion. They may also be fearful and anxious about their future should the parent die. In addition, the normal parental role model may suffer. For example, a father confined to a wheelchair will be unable to take an active part in playing games with his children. In my experience this is usually perceived as more a problem for the affected father than for his children. Nevertheless there is little doubt that children growing up in a home where a parent is physically disabled are often emotionally affected in some way, usually in childhood rather than later. Again, open and frank discussions within the family should be encouraged as far as this is possible.

Bereavement

The response to the loss of an affected child, spouse, or parent varies greatly. Though this may have been foreseen for some time, the event when it occurs is always traumatic. Some seem better able to deal with their emotions than others. But no amount of careful planning beforehand is ever entirely effective.

Table 6.1 Living with muscular dystrophy: some suggestions for consideration in discussions with professionals

Information about the disease
  Nature and outcome
  Regular follow-up
  Dietary advice
  Physiotherapy, orthoses, surgery
  Respiratory care
  Treatment
  Genetics and mode of inheritance
  Contraception, prenatal diagnosis

Psychosocial matters
  Feelings of guilt, anger, isolation
  What and when to tell
  Effects on unaffected siblings, children, partner
  Sexual problems
  Expression and sharing of emotions
  Bereavement counselling

Information about more general matters
  Address of the national muscular dystrophy group, local support group, family care
    officer, social worker, health visitor, genetic counsellor, etc. Welfare services and
    benefits
  Education, learning difficulties, residential schooling
  Holiday and babysitting schemes
  Aids and home adaptations
  Transport
  Employment opportunities

Ideally, counselling should not end with the death of the patient but should be available to all close relatives until grieving has passed. Parents and spouses may experience some sense of relief after all the years of anxiety and concern. This is all too natural and should not be a reason for feeling guilty.

Finally, for parents of affected children and for affected persons themselves, some suggestions for consideration in discussions with professionals are listed in Table 6.1. The list is clearly not exhaustive but will help focus attention on some of the more important and immediate problems where help and advice may be required.

7

Education and employment

→ Key points

♦ In planning the future education and possible employment of those with dystrophy, careful consideration has to be given to the possible effects of the disease on intellectual ability and the severity of the disease. In all cases it is important to plan ahead.

♦ In the case of Duchenne muscular dystrophy those boys who prove to be severely mentally handicapped may well require special care. Otherwise the boys' interests are usually best served by attending a normal school as long as possible.

♦ Accepting the limitations that may impair their academic performance at school and ultimately their physical capabilities, boys with Duchenne muscular dystrophy should be encouraged as much as possible to pursue subjects that they themselves find interesting and rewarding.

♦ A room at home specifically set aside for his use and interests and where he can entertain his friends is important.

♦ In the later stages, when physical disability becomes severely limiting, special schooling may be considered.

♦ In the late-onset type of dystrophy, where independent mobility can be retained for several years, adequate schooling and the careful choice of subsequent career are very important.

♦ With fitted orthoses and appropriate surgery, sedentary-type employment can be made possible for many years to come.

In all forms of muscular dystrophy careful consideration has to be given to future education and possible employment. It has been emphasized that those affected with dystrophy should be encouraged, within the limits of their disability of course, to lead as normal a life as possible and to enlarge their social contacts and circle of friends. In this way they are less likely to feel isolated and rejected. The school environment as well as employment can help a great deal in this regard. But the possibilities are very much dictated by the type of dystrophy: whether or not there is any mental impairment, the severity of the disease, and the likely degree of disability in the future. For these reasons it is helpful to consider the opportunities and problems in a severe type of dystrophy such as Duchenne muscular dystrophy, and in the late-onset, more benign types of dystrophy.

Schooling in Duchenne muscular dystrophy

There are two problems that have to be borne in mind when considering the future education of a boy with Duchenne muscular dystrophy. There is the problem of gradually increasing muscle weakness with the prospect of a wheelchair around the time he may be entering senior school, and the possibility of some degree of intellectual impairment, particularly in regard to reading skills and word comprehension (Chapter 4). However, not all boys are affected in this way and some have high IQs.

Assessment by a paediatrician or psychologist at school age will indicate whether or not there is any reduction in intelligence. For those with *severe* mental impairment (with an IQ less than 50) education in a normal school may not be feasible. Depending on the particular home circumstances it may become necessary to consider special schooling. This can be on a daily basis or be residential with the boy returning home at weekends. But there is much evidence that where there are intellectual impairments, affected boys can profit and achieve more encouraging results by attending a normal school when possible.

Most boys with Duchenne muscular dystrophy, whether intellectually compromised or not, derive most benefit from attending a normal school. Most teachers nowadays are sensitive to the particular needs of children with physical handicap and there is much to be said for visiting the school beforehand in order to discuss the situation with the head teacher and their colleagues. A school with many stairs is not going to be appropriate in future years, but increasingly educational establishments are being adapted to the needs of the disabled. Parents should convince themselves that a particular school is going to provide a happy, supportive, and sympathetic environment for their son.

Choice of subjects

In the early school years, choice of subjects is not so important. But later, boys with Duchenne muscular dystrophy should be encouraged in subjects that they enjoy and may well centre on hobbies.

It would be wrong to expect too much. Many problems affect a boy's educational ability quite apart from any inherent reduction in intellect. For instance, progressive motor disabilities make the acquisition of new skills more difficult, and even writing may become a problem. There will inevitably be more frequent absences from school in order to attend hospital for check-ups or for treatment. Boys with Duchenne muscular dystrophy often tire easily and may lack initiative and motivation. Continual encouragement is therefore important.

Attention should focus on a boy's positive abilities. Many excel in model making and some are artistically inclined. Over the years I have made a collection of paintings and drawings by patients. Their skill and ability is a frequent source of admiration by visitors to our home.

Later years

The inevitable advance of the disease makes the boy with Duchenne muscular dystrophy more vulnerable. He finds it increasingly difficult to keep up with able-bodied friends, and active participation in any sport is impossible. In fact, his school life may become much easier once he has a wheelchair. But this then means that the school must be able to deal with this situation.

There may come a point when continuation at a normal school is no longer practical and a special school for the physically disabled may then have to be considered. Some of these schools are residential, with the boy returning home at weekends. A special day or residential school may be the only solution if both parents are out all day working. There is no doubt that the mixing together and the friendships that develop between similarly affected boys is often beneficial in reducing any feelings of isolation. The alternative, of sitting for long periods at home alone in front of a television set, should never be encouraged and should be avoided if at all possible. Plans to avoid this eventuality should be made some time beforehand. Friends should be encouraged to visit. A bedroom or study, preferably on the ground floor, should be set aside for his exclusive use with TV, hi-fi, and other devices he may choose (Fig. 7.1). In this way he will have a place that he can consider his private sanctum to entertain his friends and be on his own when *he* chooses. Such arrangements become particularly important when he reaches normal school-leaving age.

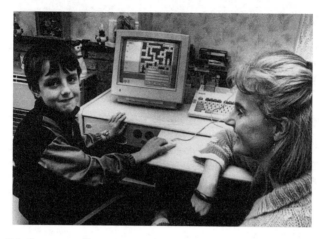

Figure 7.1 Computers offer many attractions.

Hobbies then become increasingly important and every effort should be made to encourage visitors in order to maintain his social circle.

More benign types of dystrophy

In more benign types of dystrophy, where onset may not occur until after school-leaving age and where wheelchair dependence may not be anticipated until the twenties or thirties, or even later, the problems of education and future employment are very different.

First, in most of these types of dystrophy intellect is *not* significantly impaired. In this situation every encouragement should therefore be given to a good education commensurate with the individual's abilities and interests. Secondly, as limitation of mobility can be expected later in life, this can be planned for, in terms of both education as well as possible employment opportunities.

Discussions with teachers and planning for the future are therefore essential. Few limits should be placed on what subjects might be pursued as the career opportunities for those with physical disabilities are increasing yearly.

Career opportunities

With a few obvious exceptions, such as sporting activities and those requiring physical stamina, almost any career is now open to those with physical disability.

I know of one young man with limb girdle dystrophy who nevertheless completed a course in medicine and is now a successful and internationally famous pathologist, though he is obliged to conduct his work from a wheelchair. However, it would be quite wrong to plan for a career that will ultimately prove to be physically too demanding. It all depends on the likely progression of the disease and in this regard professional advice is important.

Sedentary office-based occupations provide the best solution to the problem. Computer activities, such as graphic design or desk-top publishing, have much to commend them as they can be carried out from home. As we have seen, by fitting various orthoses as well as with appropriate surgery, many with dystrophy can hopefully look forward to employment, often for many years to come.

Motor vehicles can also be suitably modified for the disabled driver and the resulting mobility that this then permits can transform a person's life. But motor vehicle licensing authorities and insurance companies will require a doctor's medical report in order to assess the individual's ability to drive.

8

Inheritance and genetic counselling

⮞ Key points

♦ The muscular dystrophies are all genetic and may be inherited as: autosomal dominant (both sexes affected, transmitted from one generation to the next); X-linked recessive (males only affected, transmitted through females); autosomal recessive (siblings only affected).

♦ Roughly 1 in 5000 individuals in the general population is *severely* affected with some form of muscular dystrophy.

♦ Some of these are inherited as X-linked recessive traits (such as Duchenne, Becker, and Emery–Dreifuss types), some as autosomal dominant traits (facioscapulohumeral, distal, and oculopharyngeal muscular dystrophies as well as myotonic dystrophy), and some as autosomal recessive traits (most notably limb girdle dystrophy of early childhood and the congenital muscular dystrophies).

♦ By appropriate investigations including DNA studies, female carriers of X-linked dystrophies and preclinical cases of most dystrophies can now be reliably detected.

♦ Genetic counselling includes discussions of the various options available to those who consider the risks of having an affected child unacceptably high.

♦ These options include contraception, sterilization, artificial insemination by donor, ova transfer, or prenatal diagnosis. The last of these can be achieved by either transabdominal amniocentesis at about 16–18 weeks or chorion biopsy at about 11–12 weeks, the latter often now being preferred.

> ◆ Couples should never be pressurized into any course of action. They must feel free to choose the option that they see as the best and most acceptable to themselves. These decisions should never be taken lightly because the consequences can be profound and long-lasting. They should always be given the most careful consideration beforehand.

Before considering the details of how various types of muscular dystrophy are inherited, it is first useful to consider how frequent each type is in the population.

Frequency of muscular dystrophy

Knowing the number of affected persons in a population can be very useful information, for example to medical administrators in planning health care. However, as different populations are of different sizes, the number of affected persons in itself is not meaningful. Comparisons are only possible if the *total* number of individuals in a given population is also taken into account. By dividing the number of cases by the total number of individuals in a population we obtain the frequency of the disorder. There is, however, a further complication. In the case of Duchenne muscular dystrophy, for example, the frequency should ideally only relate to the number of *boys of similar age* living at the same time. To include both sexes and all ages would result in a spuriously low figure. However, in other disorders that do affect both sexes and where affected persons survive into adulthood and beyond, it is then appropriate to use the total population as the denominator in these calculations.

The frequency (or *prevalence* as this is often referred to) of various types of dystrophy has been much studied over the years, but figures in the past often varied a great deal from one study to another. This was because different types of dystrophy were sometimes erroneously lumped together and not all investigators applied the same painstaking diligence in finding cases. More recent and reliable estimates for some of the commoner types of dystrophy are given in Table 8.1. The figure given for Becker muscular dystrophy is probably too low and that for limb girdle muscular dystrophy too high because, in the past, the former was often mistakenly diagnosed as limb girdle dystrophy. In facioscapulohumeral muscular dystrophy and myotonic dystrophy the figures are only for more severely affected individuals because mildly affected cases may go undiagnosed. Including mildly affected cases, the prevalence of myotonic dystrophy may be twice the prevalence in Table 8.1. There are as yet no *reliable* figures for other types of muscular dystrophy. Furthermore, some types of

Table 8.1 Prevalence figures for some of the commoner types of muscular dystrophy

Duchenne	1 in 3500 boys
Becker	1 in 20 000 males of all ages
Limb girdle	1 in 25 000 of the total population
Facioscapulohumeral	1 in 50 000 of the total population
Myotonic dystrophy	1 in 20 000 of the total population

dystrophy may be very common in some populations (such as Fukuyama type dystrophy in Japan), but rare elsewhere. An overall figure must therefore be very approximate. But if *all* types of dystrophy are added together the overall prevalence of *severely* affected individuals in the population is probably at least 1 in 5000.

Modes of inheritance

The fact that muscular dystrophy can be familial and affect different members of the same family has been recognized for over 100 years from when Meryon noted that the disease he was studying often affected several members in a family. But the precise details as to how this Duchenne type of dystrophy was inherited was not firmly established until very much later.

As we have seen in Chapter 2, all the muscular dystrophies are *genetic*, that is, they are caused by mutations in different genes, which, in varying ways, are essential for normal muscle growth and function. But the fact that they are genetic does not necessarily mean that they are always familial and affect other members of a family. In fact they often do *not* affect other members of the family. The reason will become clear as we consider the various ways in which dystrophy can be inherited.

As we have seen in Chapter 2, each of us has 46 chromosomes, 23 derived from one parent and 23 from the other. Twenty-two of these pairs are referred to as *autosomes* and are unrelated to the sex of the individual. The remaining pair are referred to as the sex chromosomes because they determine a person's genetic sex (Fig. 8.1). These are designated as the X and Y chromosomes. Each female has two X chromosomes and each male has an X plus a small Y chromosome. It is the latter that determines that he will be male. Each egg or ovum contains a single X chromosome so that when it becomes fertilized by

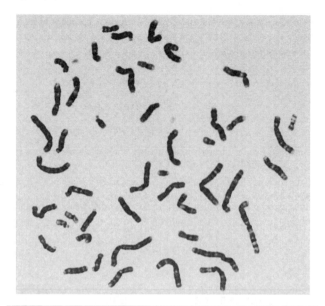

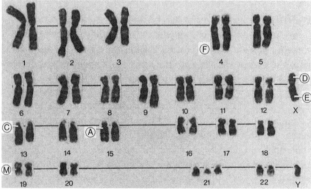

Figure 8.1 Chromosomes stained to show banding patterns by which each can be identified. *Top*: a chromosome 'spread'; *below*: the karyotype derived from the chromosome spread. The positions of the genes for various dystrophies are indicated: Duchenne and Becker (D); X-linked Emery–Dreifuss (E); two types of limb girdle of childhood (C) and (A): facioscapulohumeral (F); myotonic dystrophy (M).

an X-bearing sperm it will result in a female fetus, but if fertilized by a Y-bearing sperm it will result in a male fetus. As X- and Y-bearing sperm are produced in more or less equal numbers the number of male and female babies born is roughly equal.

Now it is helpful to imagine that each genetic trait we possess is determined by a pair of genes—one derived from our mother and the other from our father, the number of chromosomes and therefore the genes they carry being halved during the process of egg and sperm formation. If the two genes of a pair that a person inherits from his or her parents are the same then the individual is said to be *homozygous* for that gene. If the two genes are different—one being the normal gene and the other a disease-producing mutant gene—then the person is said to be a *carrier* or to be *heterozygous*. If the abnormal gene of the pair carried by the heterozygous person is 'suppressed' by the complementary normal gene then the mutant character or *trait* is said to be *recessive*. If, however, the disease-producing mutant gene is expressed and shows itself in the heterozygote, the mutant trait is said to be *dominant*. In other words, if *both* genes of a pair have to be abnormal in order to produce the disease, then the disease is said to be recessive. On the other hand, if *only one* gene of a pair needs to be abnormal to produce the disease, then the disease is said to be dominant.

No diseases are yet recognized to be due to genes on the Y chromosome. Disease genes are either located on the X chromosome (*X-linked*) or on one of the 22 pairs of autosomes. As such disease genes may be either dominant or recessive, so genetic diseases can be inherited in four possible ways: autosomal dominant, autosomal recessive, X-linked recessive, or X-linked dominant. The last possibility (X-linked dominant inheritance) has not yet been encountered in any type of muscular dystrophy. These diseases are all therefore inherited as autosomal dominant, autosomal recessive, or X-linked recessive traits.

At this point the reader might now find it less confusing and easier to follow to consider only the section on the mode of inheritance relevant to the type of dystrophy he or she is particularly interested in (see Table 8.2).

Autosomal dominant inheritance

In autosomal dominant inheritance both males and females can be affected, and a person who inherits the mutation from an affected parent will have the disease. As such a person will also have inherited a normal complementary gene (referred to as an *allele*) from the other parent, he or she will be heterozygous. In due course if this person then marries a homozygous normal

Table 8.2 Modes of inheritance of various types of muscular dystrophy. Where the disorder may *rarely* be inherited in a different manner this is indicated in brackets.

	AD	AR	XR
Duchenne and Becker			+
Emery–Dreifuss	+	(+)	+
Limb girdle			
of early childhood		+	
of later onset	+	(+)	
Facioscapulohumeral	+		
Distal	+	+	
Oculopharyngeal	+		
Congenital		+	
Myotonic dystrophy	+		

AD, autosomal dominant; AR, autosomal recessive; XR, X-linked recessive.

individual (which is usual as these are relatively rare disorders), there is a 1 in 2 (50 per cent) chance that any child will inherit the mutant gene. This is because a person passes on either of a pair of genes (alleles) to any particular offspring but never both—a fact first discovered by Gregor Mendel in pea plants over 100 years ago. (The laws of genetics apply to all living organisms.) The process will continue in each generation and it may be possible to trace the disorder back several generations (Fig. 8.2).

However, there are two points to be remembered.

1. The risk to the children of an affected person is on *average* 1 in 2. But by mere chance alone an affected parent may have several children, all of whom do not have the gene. Alternatively, such a person may be very unlucky and all the children will be affected. The risk of 1 in 2 applies to each pregnancy.

2. As many diseases inherited in this way are serious, an affected person may not survive to marry, or survive and not marry, or marry but have no children. In these circumstances it may not always be possible to trace the disease back over several generations.

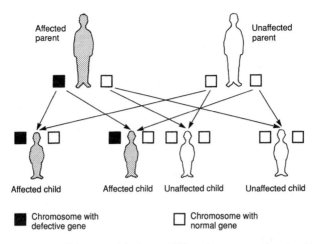

Figure 8.2 Autosomal dominant inheritance. With each pregnancy there is a 1 in 2 (50 per cent) chance of having an affected child, whatever the child's sex.

In those types of muscular dystrophy inherited as autosomal dominant traits (Table 8.2) it is usually possible to show that the disorder has been inherited from an affected parent. But where a careful clinical examination and appropriate studies (for example, DNA studies) fail to indicate any abnormality in either parent, then the affected person is likely to be the result of a *new mutation* in the egg or sperm transmitted to that particular individual. About one-third of cases of Duchenne and facioscapulohumeral muscular dystrophy are believed to result from new mutations. In which case others in the family at the time would not be at risk, although later the affected person will be at risk of having affected children. However, sophisticated DNA and other studies are beginning to show that in myotonic dystrophy, for example, new mutations are rare. It is therefore wise to assume that relatives *may* be at risk and they should be studied carefully in order to exclude the possibility that they carry the gene but do not yet have symptoms.

Risks in myotonic dystrophy

Though myotonic dystrophy is inherited as an autosomal dominant trait, the situation is more complicated because the risks to children depend on the sex of the affected parent. If the father is affected there is the usual 50 per cent risk of any of his children developing the disease in later life. But if the mother is affected the risk of losing a child through stillbirth or neonatal death is about 10 per cent, the risk of having a severely affected child with the congenital form of the disease is also 10 per cent, and the risk of having a child who will develop the disease in later life is 30 per cent. The risk of having an unaffected child is 50 per cent. Why women with myotonic dystrophy are at such a high risk of losing a baby or of having a severely affected infant is now beginning to be understood. It is due to changes in the DNA (so-called triplet expansions) at the end of the gene, which occur when the myotonic gene is transmitted by the mother in her egg, but not when transmitted by the father in his sperm.

Detection of preclinical cases

DNA tests are now becoming available for detecting *preclinical cases* of the dystrophies inherited as autosomal dominant traits. These are individuals who are heterozygous for the mutant gene, that is, they carry the mutant gene, but have not yet developed symptoms. Such tests are often requested by healthy people in affected families who are concerned that they may carry the dystrophic gene and so be at risk of having affected children.

There is a general consensus among medical scientists that testing children for a late-onset disorder such as myotonic dystrophy can lead to a great many problems. It is usually advocated that such testing be delayed until they are old enough to give consent and appreciate the implications. But clearly when an effective treatment is found, then testing could be justified at any age if this could prevent the onset of the disease later in life.

Autosomal recessive inheritance

Whereas in autosomal dominant disorders it may be possible to show that one of the parents is affected or even be able to trace the condition back through several generations, in autosomal recessive disorders this is not the case. Only brothers and sisters (siblings) can be affected. The reason is as follows. In autosomal recessive disorders, parents who carry the mutant gene appear perfectly normal. They will not know they carry the gene until they marry someone who by chance also carries the same mutant gene and they subsequently then have an affected child. Both parents may transmit either the normal gene or the mutant gene (allele) each carries to any particular child. There is then a 1 in 4 (25 per cent) chance that any child will inherit a normal gene from each parent. In this case the child will be unaffected and not carry the mutant gene. With each pregnancy of this couple there is also a 1 in 2 (50 per cent) chance of having an unaffected child who carries the mutant gene, and a 1 in 4 (25 per cent)

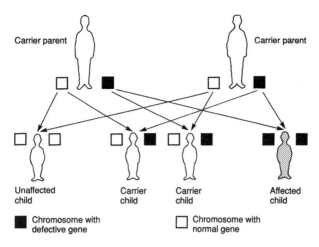

Figure 8.3 Autosomal recessive inheritance. With each pregnancy, there is a 1 in 4 (25 per cent) chance of having an unaffected child (of either sex) who does not carry the mutant gene, a 1 in 2 (50 per cent) chance of having an unaffected child who carries the mutant gene, and a 1 in 4 (25 per cent) chance of having an affected child.

chance of an affected child who has inherited a mutant gene from both parents (Fig. 8.3).

As both parents must be heterozygous and carry the same rare mutant gene (allele) this is more likely if they are blood relatives, for example cousins, who have inherited the gene from a common ancestor. In some rare autosomal recessive disorders the parents not infrequently are either first- or second-degree cousins.

If an individual with an autosomal recessive disorder survives to adulthood then he or she might be advised, as would their normal siblings who may be heterozygous, to seek a partner outside the family. It is much more likely that a relative will also carry the disease gene than some unrelated person in the population.

Quite apart from dystrophy, there are many other serious disorders that are inherited as autosomal recessive traits and we know that each one of us carries about six or so recessive genes for these disorders. It is purely *chance* that both partners come to carry the same recessive gene. Parents who therefore have a child with an autosomal recessive dystrophy should not blame each other.

X-linked recessive inheritance

This is a little more difficult to explain than autosomal inheritance but is especially important because the most common form of dystrophy (Duchenne) is inherited in this way.

As a woman has two X chromosomes, a mutation on one of her Xs will be dominated by the normal gene on the other X chromosome. She will be a heterozygous carrier who, in most cases, will be perfectly normal. When she has children she may transmit either of her Xs to her sons and daughters. Any son who inherits the X chromosome with the mutant gene will be affected as he has only one X and therefore no normal gene to counter the effects of the mutant gene. Any son who inherits her X chromosome bearing the normal gene will be normal. Thus there is a 1 in 2 (50 per cent) chance that any son she has will be affected. Similarly there is a 1 in 2 (50 per cent) chance that any daughter she has will be a carrier like herself (Fig. 8.4).

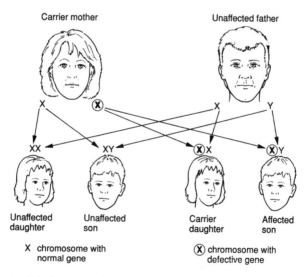

Figure 8.4 X-linked recessive inheritance. With each pregnancy in this family, where the mother is a carrier and the father is unaffected, there is a 1 in 4 (25 per cent) chance of having an unaffected daughter, a 1 in 4 (25 per cent) chance of having an unaffected son. a 1 in 4 (25 per cent) chance of having a carrier daughter, and a 1 in 4 (25 per cent) chance of having an affected son.

As boys with Duchenne muscular dystrophy do not survive to have children, the disorder in this case is transmitted by women who carry the gene. It may be transmitted in this way through unaffected females for several generations. But in about a third of families the mutation arises in the egg of a woman who does *not* carry the mutant gene. In this case it would be expected that no one else in the family would carry the gene and no one else would be affected. Such a woman might be reassured that her affected son is the result of a new mutation that should therefore not occur again in any subsequent children she may have.

However, DNA studies have now shown that the situation is more complicated than this. A woman may harbour the mutation in a whole segment of one of her ovaries and though she herself is negative for all carrier tests (see below) she is nevertheless at risk of having more than one affected son. Such women are referred to as *germline mosaics*, a mosaic referring to the fact that her ovaries are a mixture of cells, of which some have the mutant X and others do not. It is essential therefore that any mother who has had an affected son, but with no other family history of the disorder, be advised by experts in the field. It may be that in such a situation the only solution is to test the fetus in every pregnancy. This will be discussed later.

In more benign forms of X-linked muscular dystrophy (such as Becker muscular dystrophy and Emery–Dreifuss muscular dystrophy) an affected man often survives to adulthood and has children. His partner is unlikely to be a carrier and therefore as a man only transmits his Y chromosome to his sons, but his X chromosome which bears the muscular dystrophy gene to all his daughters, all his sons will be normal but all his daughters will be carriers (Fig. 8.5). His daughters will therefore be at risk of having affected sons. Thus an affected man can be sure that *none* of his children will have dystrophy but through his daughters he may have affected grandsons.

Carrier detection

For many years women in families with an X-linked muscular dystrophy, such as Duchenne dystrophy, could never be sure they were not carriers and only sure they were when they in their turn had an affected son. Then some 40 years ago it was found that about two-thirds of known carriers (women, for example, with an affected brother as well as an affected son) had significantly raised creatine phosphokinase (CPK) levels. If a woman in a family with Duchenne muscular dystrophy was tested and found to have a raised CPK level (over say 150 units) she was very likely to be a carrier, provided that the raised level could not be accounted for by other factors such as strenuous

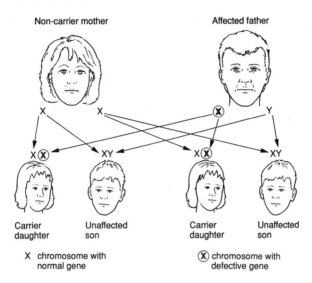

Non-carrier mother

Affected father

Carrier
daughter

Unaffected
son

Carrier
daughter

Unaffected
son

X chromosome with
   normal gene

Ⓧ chromosome with
   defective gene

Figure 8.5 X-linked recessive inheritance. With each pregnancy in this family where the father is affected, all his daughters will be carriers but all his sons will be unaffected.

exercise beforehand. Unfortunately, though this test could show that a woman was most likely to be a carrier, a normal result did not prove she was not a carrier because about a third of known carriers had CPK levels well within the normal range.

However, the situation is now much improved with the addition of various DNA tests. The latter are used to show that a mutation identified in an affected male relative is or is not present in a suspected carrier female. Problems arise, however, if there are no longer any living affected males in a family in order to identify the particular mutation in that family. These are very complicated issues that cannot be discussed in detail here. It is an area for specialists and an expert opinion should be sought in these circumstances.

Manifesting carriers

The majority of women who carry the mutant gene for Duchenne muscular dystrophy are perfectly healthy. However, it is now recognized that a small proportion (estimates vary but perhaps 1 in 20) have noticeably enlarged calves and even some proximal muscle weakness. They are referred to as manifesting carriers. Their symptoms are due to the mutant gene being expressed in a proportion of their muscle fibres. The weakness is rarely serious or progressive.

In some carriers, even in the absence of weakness, the heart may become affected. It has therefore been recommended that all carriers should know of this possibility and seek the advice of a cardiologist for potentially treatable problems. It should be emphasized, however, that the majority of carriers have no weakness at all and never have any heart problems.

The distribution and nature of the weakness can cause confusion in some cases with limb girdle muscular dystrophy and in the past such manifesting carriers were often diagnosed as having this disorder. The distinction, however, is very important because of the very different genetic risks to the children of women with these two conditions. In autosomal recessive limb girdle dystrophy there is little risk to sons or daughters of an affected female. But in the case of a manifesting carrier of X-linked Duchenne muscular dystrophy, there is of course a 1 in 2 chance of any of her sons being affected with the disease.

Fortunately, the two conditions can now be distinguished. In the manifesting carrier of Duchenne muscular dystrophy the CPK level is usually very high, the amount and distribution of dystrophin in muscle tissue are abnormal, and DNA studies may reveal a characteristic mutation associated with Duchenne dystrophy. A woman with any degree of proximal muscle weakness should seek expert advice on the possible cause and the genetic implications to her children.

Why cases may *not* be familial

We can now see why cases of muscular dystrophy that are genetic may not necessarily affect other members of a family. In autosomal dominant inheritance, a person may be affected due to a new mutation in a gene in either the egg or sperm that he or she inherited, and so no one else in the family will have been affected previously. Or, as with autosomal recessive inheritance only siblings are affected, parents may have one child with the disease and this will be the only affected person in the family.

As we have seen in X-linked recessive inheritance, except where affected males survive to have children, the disorder is inherited through carrier females who are unaffected. An affected son could be born to such a carrier, or be the result of a new mutation in a gene from an egg from a mother who is not a carrier. Either way the affected boy could be the only person with the disease in the family.

Genetic counselling

So far we have discussed how the various types of muscular dystrophy are inherited, who is likely to be affected in families, and the risk to children in such families. These are important issues that fall within the province of genetic counselling but there are many other matters that often have to be discussed as well.

Genetic counselling is essentially a process of communication between the counsellor and those who seek counselling. The term is something of a misnomer because individuals are not actually counselled, that is, advised on what to do. In fact, it should be stressed that the counsellor's role is to inform a couple about the facts and then to guide them in making a decision *that is the correct one for themselves*. There should never be any coercion on the part of the counsellor.

At one time counselling was concerned purely with medical and scientific matters: to establish a precise diagnosis, and then to communicate factual information about the disease (its nature, whether or not there is any treatment, and its course and likely outcome) and its mode of inheritance. However, more emphasis is now being given to an appreciation of the *psychological* aspects of counselling—a move away from what one might term *content-orientated* to more *person-orientated* counselling.

There are a number of reasons for this change in emphasis. First, a disabling and progressive disorder such as Duchenne muscular dystrophy has, as we have seen, profound psychological effects on the immediate family that may extend to other relatives as well. Secondly, several studies have now shown that couples sometimes opt for a course of action that may be at variance with what the counsellor may have thought 'reasonable'. Your perceptions of the disease and its risk may not be the same as the counsellor's. For example, the counsellor may feel that it would be unwise to embark on a pregnancy with the risk of producing an affected child, but this is a decision that only you can make. It is your prerogative *always provided that it is made in the full knowledge of all the facts and possible consequences*.

Timing of genetic counselling

The timing of genetic counselling is very important. It should be timed as well as tailored according to the stage in the coping process that a couple has reached (Chapter 6). It would be inappropriate and largely ignored in the early stages, and it is usually only in the later stages that counselling is likely to be accepted and effective. Any doubts about the diagnosis, and any feelings of guilt and recrimination have to be dispelled first of all.

The discussions with the counsellor should take place in private in a relaxed and quiet atmosphere. Plenty of time should be allowed for questioning. It is often helpful to go armed with a list of questions that you want answered. It is always best if both partners can be present together; there is then less likelihood of misinterpretation. Counselling can rarely be completed in a single appointment and usually requires several sessions.

Who should have genetic counselling?

The simple answer to this question is any family member who is concerned about the problem. This of course will include the parents of an affected child as well as adults with dystrophy and their partners. Furthermore, relatives who think they could be at risk may also seek counselling and often only require reassurance. If you are at all concerned about such matters then professional advice should be sought.

Options available

Genetic counselling involves not only a discussion about a particular type of dystrophy and its risks of recurrence, but also about the various options open to a couple who consider their risk of transmitting the disorder to be unacceptable. Some may decide on abstinence from sexual intercourse—a difficult decision to make but one that can provide an acceptable solution for some couples.

An alternative is to consider some form of contraception. A dread of having an affected child may well generate serious psychosexual problems for some, and effective contraception can remove a great deal of worry and lead to a more relaxed relationship between partners. But in this context expert advice is important because failure might be disastrous. For this reason *sterilization* by vasectomy for men or tubal ligation for women might have to be considered. It should be remembered, however, that though sterilization when performed on a healthy woman whose family is complete is likely to be entirely beneficial, in a young woman with a family history of Duchenne muscular dystrophy but who has no children of her own, this is a very serious decision to make and should not be taken lightly. It can have long-term psychological effects.

Artificial insemination by donor

This is a possibility where the father has a dominant form of dystrophy or if he and his partner both carry a gene for a rare autosomal recessive type of dystrophy. However, this technique has lost some of its attraction recently because of the need for very careful screening of donors in order to exclude, for example, HIV infection.

Ova transfer

This is in some ways analogous to artificial insemination. It is indicated when the mother has a dominant form of dystrophy but is able to bear children, if she is a carrier of an X-linked recessive type of dystrophy, or if she and her partner both carry a gene for a rare autosomal recessive type of dystrophy. The donor of the ova must be healthy and, if a sister for example, she must have appropriate tests to show that she is not also a carrier. Otherwise an unrelated female is best used as a donor. Ova are usually removed from the donor by a technique referred to as *laparoscopy*—a small incision is made in the abdomen, and a fine telescope is inserted through which ova can be retrieved from the ovaries. The ova are then fertilized *in vitro* with the recipient's partner's sperm. A fertilized ovum is then implanted into the recipient's uterus where it develops normally.

Pre-implantation diagnosis

Alternatively, it is now possible to remove ova from the at-risk mother and, having fertilized them with her partner's sperm, allow them to develop in culture in the laboratory until about the eight-cell stage. A single cell is then removed without damaging the rest of the conceptus. By appropriate DNA studies this can be tested to see if the abnormal mutant gene is present. If the conceptus is found to be normal it is then implanted in the uterus to complete its development. This technique is referred to as *pre-implantation diagnosis* because the diagnosis is made before the fertilized conceptus is implanted in the uterus.

Clearly these are very complicated procedures but they may prove an alternative to prenatal diagnosis. After all, not all women are able to face the prospect of prenatal diagnosis with the implication of the possibility of abortion.

Prenatal diagnosis

As the name implies, in this technique a diagnosis is made on the fetus before birth. If the fetus is shown to be affected using DNA studies, then the pregnancy can be terminated. Two methods are available for prenatal diagnosis: *transabdominal amniocentesis* and *chorion biopsy* (Fig. 8.6).

Transabdominal amniocentesis

A needle is inserted through the abdominal wall into the uterus. A small amount of fluid surrounding the fetus (*amniotic fluid*) is removed. In this fluid are cells derived from the fetus. These are separated off and then grown in a culture medium in the laboratory. After about 2 weeks there are usually sufficient cells for DNA studies on which a specific diagnosis can be made. This technique, however, is usually not possible until about 16–18 weeks of

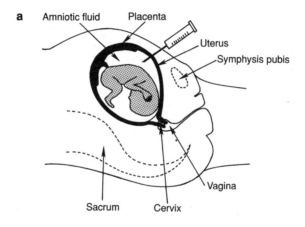

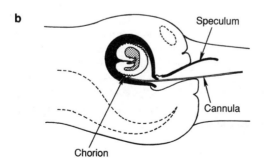

Figure 8.6 Techniques of (a) transabdominal amniocentesis and (b) chorion biopsy.

gestation and if DNA studies indicate that the fetus is affected, then termination has to take place relatively late in pregnancy. For this reason the newer method of *chorion biopsy* is often preferred.

Chorion biopsy (or chorionic villus sampling—CVS)

A flexible catheter is inserted through the cervix into the uterine cavity at about 11–12 weeks' gestation. At this stage of pregnancy, on the outside of the small amniotic sac surrounding the fetus there are small finger-like projections of cells called *chorionic villi* that are of fetal origin. A few of these are removed by the catheter and, as these villi are already living and dividing, they can often be studied directly or after only a few days in culture. The cells are then subjected to appropriate DNA studies.

As prenatal diagnosis with chorion biopsy is possible much earlier than with amniocentesis, if pregnancy termination has to be carried out it is therefore likely to be much less upsetting for the mother.

However, though both amniocentesis and chorion biopsy are safe procedures as far as the mother is concerned, both carry a small risk of precipitating an abortion. Compared with normal pregnancies of a comparable gestation, the *additional risk* is about 1 per cent for amniocentesis and about 2 per cent for chorion biopsy, though these risks depend very much on the skill and expertise of the obstetrician.

Pregnancy termination

When the result of a prenatal diagnostic test proves to be normal, the reassurance it gives is entirely beneficial. However, if the results indicate that the fetus is affected, then the consequent abortion can be psychologically very traumatic for the woman and this possibility has to be carefully considered beforehand. After an abortion a significant proportion of mothers decline to undergo the procedure again. Sensitive counselling is therefore essential both before prenatal diagnosis and subsequently after an abortion. But as Bruce Blumberg, an expert in these matters, has said 'Significant psychological trauma may be an unavoidable consequence of selective abortion, but the alternative birth of a defective child is usually accompanied by even more intense feelings of guilt and depression' (see *Psychological aspects of genetic counselling by* Emery and Pullen in the further reading section).

Counselling for individuals

From what has been implied so far it is clear that genetic counselling often involves a great deal more than discussing the nature of a disorder and risks of recurrence. It also involves the various options available if these risks are considered unacceptable. In discussing these options it is important to give careful consideration to their various advantages and disadvantages. It is important that if a couple have any reason (ethical, religious, or social) for reservations about, say, sterilization or prenatal diagnosis and abortion, they should make this clear to the counsellor from the beginning. Detailed discussion of such matters might otherwise be upsetting and not really helpful. As I have emphasized several times, these decisions rest entirely with the couple concerned.

Finally, it is very important that the genetic counsellor presents an accurate picture, even if this is depressing and disturbing, otherwise parents will be unable to make a reasoned decision about future children. A particularly difficult dilemma arises when the doctor involved in the management of a person with dystrophy also provides genetic counselling. On the one hand the doctor has to maintain an optimistic outlook, say for a child with Duchenne muscular dystrophy, and yet at the same time has to emphasize to the parents the seriousness of the disorder when discussing its possible recurrence in future children.

9

Professional and voluntary support

➲ Key points

♦ One of the most important problems in muscular dystrophy is a feeling of isolation. Help can, however, be obtained through local groups or various national organizations.

♦ Professional help is obviously important and is nowadays often based in specialist centres and units. Here the emphasis is on the comprehensive management of the disease, ideally with all the various medical, genetic, and surgical expertise being available in the one centre. Out of such centres can develop 'hospital groups' of patients and relatives.

♦ Outside the hospital environment 'patient groups' have much to commend them, not least being the opportunity they provide for social gatherings and for the sharing of worries and experiences.

♦ Finally, almost every developed country in the world now has a national organization concerned with muscular dystrophy. They act as clearing houses for information about dystrophy and maintain lists of hospital units specializing in the disease. They often provide the first point of contact for sufferers and their families.

A prevailing problem in dystrophy is a feeling of isolation. 'If only there was someone to talk to' is often heard. There is no easy solution to this problem, but there are two ways in which support can be found: through professional help and through various national organizations.

Professional help

Seven stages can be recognized in the evolution of a genetic disorder such as muscular dystrophy:

(1) positive family history;

(2) abnormality first noted;

(3) abnormality confirmed by the family doctor;

(4) diagnosis established;

(5) adaptation to the situation;

(6) progressive handicap;

(7) death and grieving.

Each of these stages presents different problems and concerns.

At stage 1 when there is a known family history of the disorder, those who feel at risk of either developing the disease themselves or of having affected children are often understandably anxious. The situation needs to be resolved and professional help and advice is essential. As we have seen, there is often a delay between the time when some abnormality is first noted and when this is confirmed by the family doctor (and not dismissed as being normal or even 'neurotic'). This period of uncertainty is very upsetting and in retrospect many parents of boys with Duchenne muscular dystrophy, as well as older people with other forms of dystrophy, look back and wonder why it took so long for their complaints to be taken more seriously. Fortunately, the situation is changing as family doctors become more aware of the possibility of muscular dystrophy and the need for specific diagnostic tests. At stage 3 the coping process begins (Chapter 6) and here it is essential that parents of affected children as well as adults with dystrophy are given every opportunity to express their anxieties and to seek professional help and advice.

During stages 4 and 5 the need for professional help continues but is usually not so compelling, except in two situations: first, at the time of having to make a decision as to whether or not to undergo surgery (Chapter 5); secondly, during the transition of boys with Duchenne muscular dystrophy from childhood to adolescence, when increased medical, social, and educational services may well be required.

Finally, bereavement is again a very traumatic time. As mentioned earlier, professional support through counselling often proves very helpful. It should not end with the death of the patient, but be available to close relatives until grieving has passed.

Specialist centres and units

There is an increasing move towards setting up regional specialist centres or units that provide *comprehensive management* for patients with muscular dystrophy. Here a team specializing in the disease is able to provide, or have local access to, all the medical and surgical expertise as well as genetic and welfare services needed.

The emphasis is on a team approach by experts in the field. Patients and their families can be seen on a regular basis and will know that they are receiving well-founded advice and treatment. Such centres, by concentrating expertise, reduce the need to travel to different hospitals for medical and other services. Often these centres are also involved in research and are therefore aware of the most recent advances. Some may also be involved in treatment trials. Those affected with dystrophy as well as their families can only benefit from these arrangements. It also means that they will meet others who have similar problems and will begin to feel less isolated.

Hospital-based groups

Groups of parents or older patients may form around a centre or unit specializing in muscular dystrophy. They may be initiated and organized by a participant and run by a nurse or social worker. These informal groups are often a useful bridge between a purely medically orientated setting and the more social setting of outside voluntary organizations.

In such groups individuals can express their anxieties and also their needs. For example, they can provide an opportunity for discussions on the various merits of different wheelchairs or used to solicit the opinion of others on the value of surgery—how it has helped them and what were the problems. They can even discuss recent developments and research findings reported in the media. Here the paediatrician or physician in charge of the clinic can be enlisted to provide answers, but in my experience parents and patients often find it easier to discuss some matters with each other and with nurses and social workers, perhaps because they feel less intimidated and therefore less inhibited.

Meetings within a hospital setting do have their value, particularly when more medical matters are an issue, but often the problems causing concern are social or even economic and then informal meetings outside are perhaps more appropriate.

Community-based groups

These informal groups initiated by parents or affected adults have much to commend them. Meeting at regular intervals in an informal way, perhaps as a coffee morning or during the evening in, for example, a school or participant's home, provide an excellent opportunity to dispel feelings of isolation. Such groups can arrange babysitting circles. These can be very valuable because the usual babysitter often feels inadequate and unable to cope with a child who is disabled. Furthermore, parents bring a competence and knowledge that would be difficult to find outside the group.

Affected adults may use such groups as the basis for a social gathering, perhaps even arranging outings and visits to places of interest.

These local groups or chapters can also become involved in fund raising for a charity organization, and in this way feel they are helping indirectly to contribute to research. They may also invite experts to address the occasional meeting and so keep up with developments in the field.

There is no doubt that many obtain a great deal of support through parent and patient groups, but not everyone finds such organizations attractive. Some would prefer to deal with matters themselves and would find participation in any association unhelpful to them personally. I have known several families like this but who, after the death of their affected son, later joined a group in order to help others.

National organizations

Almost every developed country in the world, as well as some developing countries, now has a national organization concerned with muscular dystrophy. In addition, there are also two organizations that cater for European countries as a whole: the European Alliance of Muscular Dystrophy Associations, which is largely concerned with medical and social matters, and the European Neuromuscular Centre (ENMC), concerned with research into muscular dystrophy and related disorders. These various organizations and their addresses are listed at the end of the book. They act as 'clearing houses' for information about muscular dystrophy. The Muscular Dystrophy Campaign of Great Britain, for example, produces a series of leaflets on the dystrophies. Each deals with a specific disease, covering its clinical features and mode of inheritance. There are also leaflets on particular topics such as physiotherapy, weight control, care of respiratory function, equipment and aids, and the surgical correction of spinal deformity. Many organizations also produce and circulate newsletters at regular intervals. They also maintain lists of hospital units specializing in dystrophy to which a patient can be referred for treatment. The ENMC, for example, has produced a useful booklet called *Who's who in neuromuscular disorders*.

Importantly, these organizations often provide the first point of contact for sufferers from muscular dystrophy and their families. Through their fund-raising activities, they raise significant sums of money for research, which is channelled through various hospitals, universities, and research organizations. Without such support, and the encouragement of these organizations, it is very doubtful if any significant advances in research into muscular dystrophy would have taken place.

10

The future

Until a few years ago, there seemed little chance of ever really understanding what caused muscular dystrophy, let alone finding a cure. Because the muscle histology (Chapter 3) in each of these disorders was so similar, there was a general feeling that they all might therefore share the same cause.

At first it was thought they might be due to some defect in the blood supply to the muscle. This was not a new idea because Duchenne had entertained a similar notion over 100 years ago, but the proponents never managed to produce any really convincing evidence. Then in 1970, based largely on electromyographic work, the idea that dystrophy might be due to a defect in the muscle's nerve supply came into vogue. It was suggested that perhaps some hypothetical substance that normally passed down a nerve to 'feed' the muscle (the so-called *trophic factor*) was missing or defective in muscular dystrophy. A great deal of research effort was expended on this idea, but when the original nerve studies on which it was based were seriously questioned the whole concept was thrown into doubt.

However, in the mid-1970s Allen Roses and his colleagues at Duke University, North Carolina, presented biochemical evidence of a possible defect in the *membrane* of various tissues in dystrophy and not just in muscle. These findings had instant appeal for many investigators working in the field because, since the dystrophies are genetic, one might therefore expect the defect to be also expressed in tissues other than muscle. Many of the subsequent abnormalities reported by different groups, for example in red-cell membranes, often proved controversial, but there was little doubt that a defect in the muscle fibre membrane did exist and would explain a great deal, including the leak of creatine kinase into the circulation (Chapter 3).

Then an entirely new approach to understanding the basic defects in genetic disorders began to be pursued by molecular geneticists. This approach involves first locating a defective mutant gene to a particular chromosome, and then to a particular place (its *locus*) on the chromosome. By a number of ingenious techniques the gene is then isolated and cloned and its protein product identified. With this new technology it thus became possible to identify the specific defects in various genetic disorders.

This approach resulted in the successful location of the gene for Duchenne muscular dystrophy to the short arm of the X chromosome (at a position referred to as Xp21). Subsequently Becker muscular dystrophy was shown to be due to a different mutation but at the same gene locus. Finally in 1987 the responsible gene was cloned and its protein product identified and named dystrophin. This protein is now known to be important in the structure of the muscle cell membrane (Table 10.1). This was the result of truly international efforts involving, among others, Kay Davies of Oxford, Ron Worton of Toronto, Lou Kunkel of Boston, and Eric Hoffman of Pittsburgh, and their associates. One important paper on the subject published in the scientific journal *Nature* listed no less than 75 co-authors from all over the world!

In some forms of dystrophy (notably facioscapulohumeral dystrophy and myotonic dystrophy) the disease-causing genes have been located but their protein products not yet characterized. We therefore still do not know the basic cause of these disorders. But now with ever-improving technology, answers will no doubt soon be found, perhaps even as this book is being written.

Though an effective treatment has not yet been found for Duchenne muscular dystrophy, we are much closer to this now than at any other time in the past.

Table 10.1 Some landmarks in the history of Duchenne muscular dystrophy (DMD) and Becker muscular dystrophy (BMD)

Nineteenth century	DMD recognized as a specific disorder
1955	BMD recognized as a specific disorder
1959–60	Serum CPK first shown to be raised in patients and carriers
1978–83	DMD gene located on the X chromosome (at position Xp21)
1983–84	BMD also located at Xp21
1985	DNA markers available for carrier detection and prenatal diagnosis
1987–88	Gene cloned and protein product identified (dystrophin)
1990–	Gene therapy studies in animals. Protocols for similar studies in human dystrophy considered
1999–	Stem cell therapeutic studies in animals

This may well prove possible using a drug, perhaps designed for the purpose by pharmacologists, which specifically influences or interrupts the sequence of events between the deficiency of dystrophin and the development of weakness. Alternatively, some form of gene therapy may prove a more effective approach. If so, when this day comes and gene therapy is shown to work in Duchenne muscular dystrophy, the same approach will no doubt also be applicable to other dystrophies. The future now looks more hopeful and encouraging than at any other time in the history of muscular dystrophy.

Living with muscular dystrophy

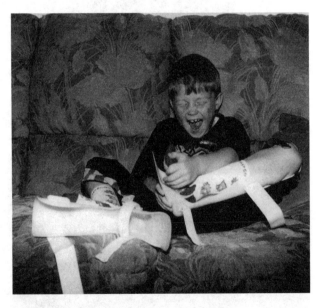

Even putting on splints can be fun.

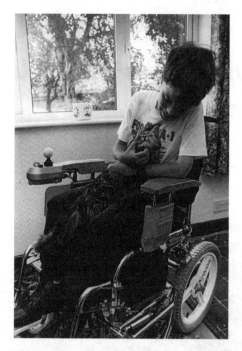

The companionship of a pet is often very important.

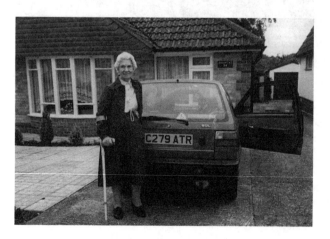

An adapted car means greater independence.

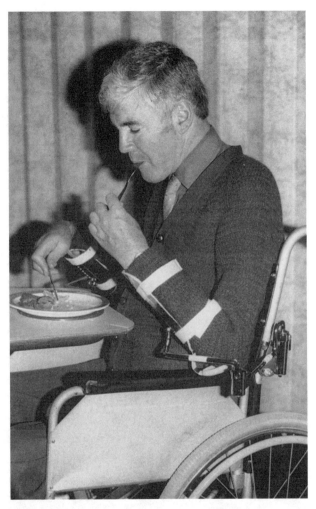

Quite simple devices can often make everyday living much easier.

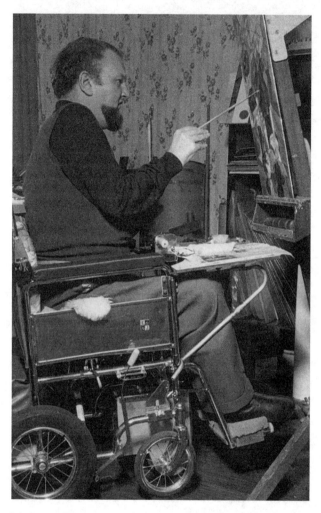

Painting can be a very rewarding pastime for the disabled.

Appendix 1

Further reading and information

The Muscular Dystrophy Campaign (MDC) is the only national charity focusing on all muscular dystrophies and related muscle diseases. It has pioneered the search for treatments and cures for nearly 50 years, and is dedicated to improving the lives of those people affected by providing practical and emotional care and support, funding world-class research to find effective treatments and cures, campaigning to raise awareness and increase the independence of people with muscle disease.

Information and support service is free to use. Call 0800 652 6352 between 9am and 5pm, Monday to Friday, to get any information you might need, or visit the website (www.muscular-dystrophy.org).

The MDC relies almost entirely on voluntary donations to fund its groundbreaking and vital work.

The following are texts that deal in greater detail with some of the topics discussed in this little book.

Reference texts which deal with most aspects of muscular dystrophy

Bertorini TE (Ed.) (2002) *Clinical evaluation and diagnostic tests for neuromuscular disorders*. Butterworth–Heinemann, London.

Dubowitz V (1995) *Muscle disorders in childhood* (2nd edn). W.B. Saunders, London.

Emery AEH (Ed.) (1998) *Neuromuscular disorders: clinical and molecular genetics*. John Wiley, Chichester.

Emery AEH (Ed.) (2001) *The muscular dystrophies*. Oxford University Press.

Karpati G. Hilton-Jones D, Griggs RS (Eds.) (2001) *Disorders of voluntary muscle* (7th edn). Cambridge University Press.

Swash M, Schwartz MS (1997) *Neuromuscular disorders* (3rd edn). Springer-Verlag, London.

Monographs on specific disorders

Brown SC, Lucy JA (Eds) (1997) *Dystrophin: gene, protein and cell biology.* Cambridge University Press.

Emery AEH, Muntoni F (2003) *Duchenne muscular dystrophy* (3rd edn). Oxford University Press.

Emery AEH, Emery M (1995) *The history of a genetic disease: Duchenne muscular dystrophy.* Royal Society of Medicine Press, London.

Fukuyama Y, Osawa M, Saito K (Eds) (1997) *Congenital muscular dystrophies.* Elsevier, Oxford.

Harper PS (2001) *Myotonic dystrophy* (3rd edn). W.B. Saunders, London.

Muscular Dystrophy Association of America. (1998) *Journey of love – a parent's guide to Duchenne muscular dystrophy.* MDAA, Tucson, AZ.

Texts which deal with particular topics relevant to muscular dystrophy

General guidance

Thompson CE (1999) *Raising a child with a neuromuscular disorder.* Oxford University Press.

Bereavement

Lake T. (1984, 1992) *Living with grief.* Sheldon Press/Abingdon Press, London.

Genetic counselling

Emery AEH, Pullen I (Eds) (1984) *Psychological aspects of genetic counselling.* Academic Press, London.

Harper PS (1998) *Practical genetic counselling* (5th edn). Wright, London.

Physiotherapy

Hemmings L (2006) *Physiotherapy management of Duchenne muscular dystrophy.* Muscular Dystrophy Campaign, London.

Prenatal diagnosis

Brock D, Rodeck C, Ferguson-Smith M (Eds) (1992) *Prenatal diagnosis and screening*. Churchill Livingstone, Edinburgh.

Sexual matters

The Family Planning Association, 50 Featherstone Street, London ECIY 8QU, has a telephone helpline (0845 122 8690) and provides information on all aspects of family planning and sexual and reproductive health. A helpful website is Disability Now (http://www.disabilitynow.org.uk).

Housing adaptations

Harpin P (2006) *Muscular dystrophy adaptations manual* (2nd edn). Muscular Dystrophy Campaign, London.

Books about the disease written by patients or their relatives

Journey of love (1998) Published by the Muscular Dystrophy Association of America, this gives a very full list of books by and about people with muscular dystrophy.

Pettenuzzo B, Gwatkin T (1989) *I have muscular dystrophy*. Franklin Watts, London.

Wilson B (1996) *Brenton's story*. Children's Society, London.

Journals

Research developments are often reported in medical, paediatric, neurological, or scientific journals. Journals in English specifically concerned with neuro-muscular disorders are:

Muscle and Nerve (published monthly by John Wiley, New York and Chichester).

Neuromuscular Disorders (published monthly by Elsevier, Oxford).

Basic and Applied Myology (published four times a year by Unipress, Padova, Italy).

See also:

Orto AED, Marinelli RP (1995) *Encyclopedia of disability and rehabilitation*. Macmillan, London.

Appendix 2

Patient support groups

The Muscular Dystrophy Campaign (MDC)is a registered charity and not only provides funds for research into the causes and treatment of muscular dystrophy, but also provides much useful information for patients and their families.

Muscular Dystrophy Campaign

61 Southwark Street
London SE1 0HL
Tel: 020 78034800
Fax: 020 74013495
Email: info@muscular-dystrophy.org
Web: www.muscular-dystrophy.org

There are a number of support groups concerned with specific conditions.

Becker muscular dystrophy

Becker United
Email: tjd.davies@ntlworld.com
Web: http://www.beckerunited.com

Duchenne muscular dystrophy

Duchenne Family Support Group
78 York Street
London W1H 1DP
Tel: 0870 2411857
Helpline: 0870 6061604
Email: info@dfsg.org.uk
Web: http://www.dfsg.org.uk

PPUK (Parent Project UK)

Epicentre

41 West Street

London E11 4LJ

Tel: 020 85569955

Email: info@ppuk.org

Web: http://www.ppuk.org

Facioscapulohumeral muscular dystrophy

FSH Support Group

8 Caldecote Gardens

Bushey Heath

Hertfordshire WD23 4GP

Tel: 020 89507500

Web: http://www.fsh-group.org

Mitochondrial myopathies

Mitochondrial Myopathies

3 Home Farm Cottages

Yearby

Nr Redcar

Cleveland TS11 8HQ

Tel: 01642 480953

Email: mitolinksuk@aol.com

Web: http://www.communigate.co.uk/ne/mitolinks

Myotonic dystrophy

Myotonic Dystrophy Support Group

35A Carlton Hill

Nottingham NG4 1BG

Answerphone: 0115 9875869

Email: mdsg@tesco.net

Web: http://www.mdsguk.org

Oculopharyngeal muscular dystrophy

OPMD Support Group

13 Helmsley Road

Leeds LS16 5JA

Tel: 0113 2753048

Web: http://www.opmdsupport.co.uk

There are several other support groups concerned with other forms of muscle disease. Details are available from the Muscular Dystrophy Campaign.

Appendix 3

Muscular dystrophy associations and groups in various countries

Australia

Muscular Dystrophy Association of New South Wales

Locked Bag 9932, Beaconsfield, NSW 2014

Tel.: 61 (0)296979111

Fax: 61 (0)296979092

Email: info@mdansw.org

Web: http://www.mdansw.org.au

Muscular Dystrophy Association Inc. South Australia

GPO Box 414, Adelaide, SA 5001

Tel.: 61 (0)882345266

Fax: 61 (0)882345866

Email: info@mdasa.org.au

Web: http://www.mdasa.org.au

Muscular Dystrophy Association of Western Australia

PO Box 328, West Perth, WA 6872

Tel.: 61 (0)893822700

Fax: 61 (0)893463487

Email: mda@cyllene.uwa.edu.au

Web: http://www.mdawa.asn.au

Muscular Dystrophy Association Queensland

Locked Bag 3000, Spring Hill, QLD 4004
Tel.: 61 (0)730161800
Fax: 61 (0)738312666
Web: http://www.mdaq.com.au

Muscular Dystrophy Association Ltd

PO Box 2200, North Melbourne
Victoria 3051
Tel.: 61 (0)393209555
Fax: 61 (0)393209595
Email: bms@mda.org.au
Web: http://www.mda.org.au

Belgium

Assoc Belge contre les Maladies Neuro-Muscularies (ASBL)

Alléé des champs de Blé 64
7033 Mons (Cuesmes)
Tel.: 32 (0)65841844
Email: info@abmm.be
Web: http://www.abmm.be

Flemish Muscular Disorders Association

Vlaamse Vereniging Neuromusculaire Aandoeningen (NEMA)
Nadine Albergs
Helgbeekplein 1 bus 25
3500 Hasselt
Tel.: 32 (0)11723187
Email: sekretariaat@nema.be
Web: http://www.nema.be

Brazil
Associacão de Amigos dos Portadores de Distrofia Muscular (AADM)

Tel.: 55 (16)39193028

Web: http://www.aadm.com.br

Canada
Muscular Dystrophy Association of Canada

2345 Yonge Street, Suite 900

Toronto

Ontario M4P 2E5

Tel.: 1 8666872538

Fax: 1 4164887523

Email: info@muscle.ca

Web: http://www.muscle.ca

Croatia
Union of Muscular Dystrophy Societies of Croatia

Nova Ves 44, 10000 Zagreb

Tel.: 385 14666849

Email: sddh@zg.t-com.hr

Web: http://www.sddh.hr

Cyprus
The Cyprus Institute of Neurology and Genetics

PO Box 23462

1683 Nicosia

Tel.: 357 22358600

Web: http://www.cing.ac.cy

Czech Republic
Asociace muskulárnich dystrofiku v CR

Petyrkova 1953/24

Praha 4 Chodov 148 00

Czech Republic

Tel.: 420 7933777

Fax: 420 7933777

Email: amd@cmail.cz

Web: http://www.md-cz.org

Denmark
Muskelsvindfonden

Kongsvag Allé 23

DK-8000 Århus C

Tel.: 45 89482222

Fax: 45 39622205

Email: mrf@muskelsvindfonden.dk

Web: http://www.muskelsvindfonden.dk

Estonia
Estonian Association of Muscular Disorders

Email: els@els.ee

Web: http://www.els.ee

Finland
Lihastautiliittory

Läntinen Pitkäkatu 35

20100 Turku

Tel.: 358 (02)2739700

Fax: 358 (02)2739701

Email: lihastautiliitto@lihastautiliitto.fi

Web: http://www.lihastautiliitto.fi

France
Association Française contre les Myopathies (AFM)

1 Rue de l'Internationale

BP 59

91002 Evry Cedex

Tel.: 33 169472828

Web: http://www.afm-france.org

Germany
Deutsche Gesellschaft fur Muskellkranke eV

Im Moos 4

79112 Freiburg

Tel.: 49 7665944720

Fax: 49 7665944720

Email: info@dgm.org

Web: http://www.dgm.org

Greece
MDA Hellas

Email: info@mdahellas.gr

Web: http://www.mdahellas.gr

India
Muscular Dystrophy Association India

c/o Molecular Diagnostic Facility

Sundaram Medical Foundation

Dr Rangarajan Memorial Hospital

Shanthi Colony, 4th Avenue

Anna Nagar, Chennai 600 040

Tel.: 91 4426268844 Ext. 349 or 350

Fax: 91 4426284257

Email: ranil@vsnl.com

Email: wiswanathan@vsnl.com

Web: http://www.mdaindia.org

Ireland
Muscular Dystrophy Ireland (MDI)

71–72 North Brunswick Street

Dublin 7

Tel.: 353 (0)18721501

Fax: 353 (0)18724482

Email: info@mdi.ie

Web: http://www.mdi.ie

Italy
Unione Italiana Lotta alla Distrofia Muscolare—Direzione Nazionale

Via P.P. Vergerio

19-35126 Padova

Tel.: 39 (0)498021001 or (0)49757361

Fax: 39 (0)49757033

Web: http://www.uildm.org

Japan
Japan Muscular Dystrophy Association Corp.

2-2-2 Nishi-Waseda, Shinjuko-Ku
Tokyo 162-0051
Tel.: 81 352732930
Fax: 81 332087030
Web: http://www.jmda.or.jp

Jordan
Al-Hussein Society for the Habilitation/Rehabilitation of the Physically Challenged

PO Box 5102
Amman 11183
Tel.: 962 (0)65817598/99
Fax: 962 (0)65817613
Email: ahsrehab@wanadoo.jo
Web: http://www.alhusseinrehab.org.jo

Kosovo
Muscular Dystrophy Associations of Kosovo

Str Ardian Krasnici N:6/22
Priština, Kosovo
Tel.: (0)38247721 or (0)44222659
Email: gimi_mda@yokso.com

Malta
Muscular Dystrophy Group of Malta and European Alliance of Neuromuscular Disorders Associations (EAMDA)

4 Gzira Road, Gzira GZR 04, Malta
Tel.: 356 21346688
Fax: 356 21318024
Email: mdg@mdgmalta.com *or* eamda@hotmail.com
Web: http://www.mdgmalta.com or www.eamda.net

Mexico
Sociedad Mexicana de la Distrofia Muscular AC

Calz. México Xochimilco No. 289
Col. Arenal de Guadalope
Delagación Tlalpan, C.P. 14389
Tel.: 52 5559991000 Ext. 13230
Email: distrofhiamx@yahoo.com.mx
Web: http://www.cnr.gob.mx/SMDM

Nepal
Muscular Dystrophy Foundation-Nepal (MDF-Nepal)

GPO Box 8975 EPC 697
Lalitpur, Kathmandu
Tel.: 977 15546984
Email: info@mdfnepal.wlink.com.np
Web: http://www.mdfnepal.org.np

The Netherlands
Vereniging Spierziekten Nederland

Lt Gen van Heutslaan 6
3743 JN, Baarn
Tel.: 31 (0)355480480
Email: vsn@vsn.nl
Web: http://www.vsn.nl

New Zealand
New Zealand Muscular Dystrophy Association

PO Box 16–238, Sandringham, Auckland 1030
New Zealand
Tel.: 64 (0)98150247
Fax: 64 (0)98157260
Email: info@mda.org.nz
Web: http://www.mda.org.nz

Norway
Norway Muscular Dystrophy Association

Foreningen for Muskelsyke
Bergsalléen 21
0854 Oslo
Tel.: 47 23215450
Email: ffm@ffm.no
Web: http://www.ffm.no

Peru
Asociacion de Distrofia Muscular del Peru—ADM Peru

Av. Del Ejercito 660-F
Miraflores, Lima 18
Peru
Tel.: 51 1226322/6472
Fax: 51 12413140
Email: admperu@ec-red.com
Web: http://www.admperu.cjb.net

Poland
Polskie Towarzystar Corób Nerwowo-miesnionych

Ul.Sw. Bonifacego 10
02-914 Warszawa
Tel/fax: 48(0)226427507
Email: ptchnm@idn.org.pl
Web: http://www.idn.org.pl/tzchm

Romania

Asociatia Distroficilor Muscular din Romania

707085-Lunca Cetatuii B1.65

Tr. II, parter, Ap 3

Com. Ciurea

Judetul lasi

Tel/fax: 40 232296075

Email: admr_filialaiasi@yahoo.com

Web: http://www.admiasi.3x.ro

Singapore

Muscular Dystrophy Association Singapore (MDAS)

9 Bishan Place #06-01

Junction 8

Singapore 579837

Tel.: 65 62596933

Fax: 65 62596911

Email: mdas@mdas.org.sg

Web: http://www.mdas.org.sg

Slovakia

Organizácia Muskulárnych Dystrofikov v Slovenskej Republike

Banselova 4

821 04 Bratislava 2

Tel.: 421 (0)243411686

Tel/fax: 421 (0)243410474

Web: http://www.omdvsr.sk

Slovenia
Drustvo distrofikov Slovenije

p.p. 2618, Linhartova 1/111
1001 Ljubljana
Tel.: 386 (0)14720500
Web: http://www.drustvo-distrofikov.si

South Africa
Muscular Dystrophy Foundation of South Africa

National Office, PO Box 1535
Pinegowrie 2123
Tel/fax: 27 (011)7897634
E-mail: national@mdsa.org.za
Web: http://www.mdsa.org.za

Spain
Federacion Española de Enfermedades Neuro Musculares (Federacion ASEM)

C. Jordi de Sant Jordi
26–28 Bajos
08027 Barcelona
Tel.: 34 934516544
Fax: 34 934083695
Email: asem15@suport.org
Web: http://www.asem-esp.org

Sweden
Swedish Association of Neurologically Disabled

Box 49 084
S-100 28 Stockholm
Tel.: 46 (0)86777010
Email: nhr@nhr.se
Web: http://www.nhr.se

The Swedish National Association for Disabled Children

St Eriks Gatan 44

S-104 20 Stockholm

Tel.: 46 (0)86777300

Email: info@riks.rub.se

Web: http://www.rbu.se

Switzerland

Association de la Suisse Romande et Italienne contre les Myopathies (ASRIM)

12 ch. de la Traverse 12

CP 179

CH-1170 Aubonne

Tel.: 41 (0)218087411

Fax: 41 (0)21808 8111

E-mail: info@asrim.ch

Web: http://www.asrim.ch

Schweizerische Gesellschaft fur Muskelkranke (SGMK)

Kanzleistrasse 80

8004 Zurich

Switzerland

Tel.: 41 (0)442458030

Fax: 41 (0)44 2458031

Email: info@muskelkrank.ch

Web: http://www.muskelkrank.ch

United Kingdom
Muscular Dystrophy Campaign

61 Southwark Street
London SE1 0HL
Tel.: 0800 6526352
Email: info@muscular-dystrophy.org
Web: http://www.muscular-dystrophy.org

United States of America
Muscular Dystrophy Association—USA

National Headquarters
3300 E. Sunrise Drive
Tucson, AZ 85718
Tel.: 1 8003444863
Email: mda@mdausa.org
Web: http://www.mdausa.org

Yugoslavia
Yugoslavia Muscular Dystrophy Association

Udruzenje Distroficara Jugoslavije
Kragujevac, ul. Kosovska b.b.
Tel.: 381 (0)34305875
Fax: 381 (0)34305876
Email: kragujevac@udruzenjedistroficara.org.yu
Web: http://www.udruzenjedistroficara.org.yu

Glossary

This glossary gives definitions of scientific terms; in some cases the definitions given refer *only to their use in this book*. Words in italic are defined in the glossary.

action potential: electrical activity produced by contracting muscle fibres

alleles: alternate forms of the same gene—the normal and its mutant(s)

amino acids: small organic compounds that are the building blocks of *proteins*

amniocentesis: procedure for removing a small amount of *amniotic fluid* for *prenatal* diagnosis

amniotic fluid: fluid that surrounds the fetus in the womb (uterus)

anterior tibial: at the outer side of the front of the shin bone or *tibia*

artificial insemination by donor: insemination of a woman with sperm from a donor other than her partner

autosome: any chromosome other than the sex chromosomes

biopsy: removal of a small amount of tissue (usually muscle) for examination

cardiac muscle: heart muscle

carrier: an individual who has inherited a normal gene from one parent and a particular abnormal gene (*allele*) from the other; also referred to as a *heterozygote*

cataracts: opacities in the lens of the eye, sometimes also referred to as lenticular opacities

catheter: a long slender flexible tube

chorion: outer layer of cells which cover the developing embryo

chorion biopsy: removal of fetal *chorionic villi* for prenatal diagnosis, sometimes also referred to as chorionic villus sampling—CVS

chorionic villi: finger-like projections of the *chorion*

chromosomes: thread-like bodies within the *nucleus* that stain with particular dyes; they contain the *genes*

clone: all the cells derived from a single cell by repeated division and therefore all having the same genetic constitution

conceptus: the fertilized ovum and the embryo into which it develops

congenital: present at birth (or soon afterwards)

consanguinity: the genetic relatedness between individuals of the same family, such as cousins

contractures: shortening of muscles usually due to prolonged immobility (though not in Emery–Dreifuss dystrophy for example), which results in the associated joints becoming fixed and no longer able to move freely

coping process: the psychological sequence of events that follow any stressful situation

CPK: abbreviation for creatine phosphokinase, sometimes shortened to CK (creatine kinase), a muscle enzyme important in muscle contraction

creatine kinase: see CPK

CT: abbreviation for computed tomography, a radiographic diagnostic technique for producing images of internal body organs, including muscle

CVS: see *chorion biopsy*

cytoplasm: the substance of the cell in which the *nucleus* and *mitochondria* are located

diploid: the number of *chromosomes* in the cells of the human body (46); each cell contains two sets of chromosomes, one set derived from each parent

diplopia: double vision

disorder: another term for disease

distal: part of the limb most distant from the trunk (e.g. forearms and hands, lower legs and feet)

DNA: deoxyribonucleic acid—the chemical basis of genes in which there is coded information for synthesizing *proteins*

dominant: an abnormal gene that is expressed in the *heterozygote*

dysphagia: difficulty in swallowing

dystrophin: a protein associated with the *membrane* surrounding each *muscle fibre*, which is absent in Duchenne muscular dystrophy and abnormal in Becker muscular dystrophy

ECG (or EKG): abbreviation for electrocardiogram, a non-invasive method for studying the function of the heart

EMG: abbreviation for electromyogram, an electrical test used in diagnosing muscular dystrophies

endocrine glands: glands that secrete substances into the blood, which then affect other organs (e.g. thyroid gland)

enzymes: particular proteins in the cell responsible for chemical reactions

familial: a term for a *trait* or disease which can affect several members of the same family

gametes: sperm and ova

gene: part of the DNA molecule that is responsible for synthesizing proteins

gene marker: a small segment (sequence) of DNA that is used to identify a mutant gene in an individual or trace its inheritance within a family

gene probe: a small segment (sequence) of DNA that is identical with part or all of a gene

gene therapy: treatment of inherited disease by the addition or substitution of a normal gene

genetic: any characteristic or *trait* that is inherited

genome: all the genes in a cell

germ cell: a sex cell

germline mosaic: the presence in the ovary of two different populations of cells

glycoproteins: a group of proteins which, with other proteins including *dystrophin*, are associated with and maintain the integrity of the muscle fibre *membrane*

Gower's sign: pressing on the thighs in order to straighten up

graft rejection: the rejection of a transplanted tissue or organ due to the host's *immune response* to the 'foreign' material

haploid: the number of *chromosomes* in each of the *gametes* (23 in humans)

heart block: a defect in the conducting system of the heart that results in abnormal slowing of the heart rate

heterozygote: an individual who has inherited a normal gene from one parent and a particular abnormal genes (*allele*) from the other; also referred to as a *carrier*

histochemistry: the microscopic chemical study of tissues such as muscle

histology: the microscopic study of tissues such as muscle

homozygote: an individual who has inherited a particular allele from *both* parents (two identical abnormal genes in a homozygous affected individual)

humerus: the upper arm bone

hypoxia: low oxygen level in the blood

immune response: the response by the body to 'foreign' material (transplant or infection) that is thereby destroyed

in utero: literally, in the uterus

in vitro: literally, in glass, meaning in the laboratory; thus, in *vitro* fertilization is the fertilization of an egg by a sperm in a test tube in the laboratory

ion: an electrically charged atom

isotonic: a solution of salts of the same composition as the body fluids

karyotype: a photomicrograph of an individual's chromosomes arranged in pairs in a standard manner, from the largest (number 1) down to the smallest (number 22) autosomes and the two sex chromosomes

laparoscopy: insertion of a fine telescopic tube into the abdomen in order to visualize organs such as the ovaries

lenticular (lens) opacities: see *cataracts*

leucocyte: a white blood cell

limb girdle: hips and shoulders

locus: the location of a gene on a chromosome

lordosis: exaggerated forward curvature of the lower back

macrophage: a cell in diseased muscle that consumes necrotic fibres

manifesting carrier: a female *carrier* of an *X-linked* muscular dystrophy who has some weakness

meiosis: the process of cell division in the sex cells that results in *haploid gametes*

membrane: surrounding outer layer

mitochondria: minute structures or organelles within the cell concerned with the production of energy

mitosis: the process of division in the body cells

molecular genetics: the study of genes at the submicroscopic level

mosaic: two different populations of cells in the same tissue (e.g. ovary) of an individual

MRI: abbreviation for magnetic resonance imaging (*see* CT)

muscle fibre: the basic unit of muscle tissue; formed by the fusion of groups of muscle cells each having one *nucleus* to produce muscle fibres with many nuclei

mutation: changed and abnormal gene; sometimes used to described an individual with a genetic abnormality not present in the genes of either parent

myoglobin: oxygen-carrying *protein* of muscle

myometer: instrument used to measure muscle strength

myopathic: originating in the muscle

myopathy: any disease of muscle

myotonia: delayed relaxation after muscle contraction

necrosis: literally, death; a descriptive term for the microscopic changes seen in muscle fibres in muscular dystrophy

neurogenic: originating in the nervous system

nucleus: the structure within the cell that contains the *chromosomes*

ocular: relating to the eye

orthoses: devices or aids to prevent or correct deformities

pathogenesis: the development of the disease process

pectoral: in the shoulder region

pelvic: in the hip region

peroneal: more or less synonymous with *anterior tibial*

pharyngeal: relating to the *pharynx*

pharynx: the upper part of the airways, at the back of the throat

placebo: an inactive compound that closely resembles an active drug

preclinical diagnosis: diagnosis of a genetic disorder *before* there are any symptoms of the disorder

pre-implantation diagnosis: diagnosis of a disorder in the fertilized *conceptus* before it becomes implanted into the uterus

prenatal: literally, before birth

prevalence: frequency of a disorder in a population

prognosis: probable course and outcome of a disease

promoter: a segment (sequence) of DNA that 'turns on' an associated *gene*

proteins: large molecules, composed of *amino acids*, which are essential components of the body; they include *enzymes*

proximal: part of the limb closest to the trunk (e.g. upper arms, shoulders, thighs, and hips)

pseudohypertrophy: enlargement of muscles (usually the calves), which can occur in dystrophy

ptosis: drooping of the eyelids

recessive: an abnormal gene that is only expressed in the *homozygote*

sarcolemma: two-layered outer membrane of muscle fibres

scapula: the shoulder blade

scapular: around the shoulder

scoliosis: curvature of the spine to one side

sex chromosomes: the pair of non-*autosomal* genes which determine an individual's sex (XX in the female, XY in the male)

sex-linked: a gene on the X chromosome

sibling (or sib): brother or sister

skeletal muscles: those muscles that move joints

slit lamp: an instrument used by ophthalmologists to examine the lens of the eye

smooth muscle: involuntary muscles of the gut and blood vessels

somatic cells: cells of the body other than the sex cells (*gametes, germ cells*)

Southern blot: a method of transferring DNA fragments to a nitrocellulose filter where they can be tested using a *gene marker* or *gene probe*

stem cell: a cell capable of dividing and growing into different tissues of the body

steroids: a group of drugs that have a wide range of uses in medicine, including the suppression of the *immune response* (e.g. after a tissue transplant)

syndrome: the complex of signs and symptoms that occur together in any particular disorder

talipes: turning in of the sole of the foot

tibia: shin bone

tibial: relating to the *tibia*

tracheostomy: insertion of a tube (airways) into the upper trachea (windpipe)

trait: an inherited characteristic

ultrasound: sound waves above hearing frequencies, used to study internal body organs (e.g. muscle structure, the position of the placenta, and the fetus *in utero*)

vector: a virus used to carry a human gene

venepuncture: removal of a blood sample from a vein

X-linked: gene on the X chromosome (synonymous with *sex linked*)

Index